"Aging Deliberately … so much common sense, so much help, so much fun. Thanks Steve and Tom."

"This book is a joy! I found myself nodding in agreement, smiling, and making plans for change and growth as I read…."

"*Aging Deliberately* is inspirational. Thanks to Steve and Tom I am ready to get out of my chair, clean out the fridge, and get back to really living my life again."

"Steve's book makes it all so clear: This aging business really is all about attitude, action, and loving yourself."

"I have read each of Steve's books (deliberately). Always plenty of great, helpful information without a lecture. I am anxiously awaiting the next one!"

"I have read dozens of articles and books about aging. What Tom and Steve have come up with is the most comprehensive and helpful approach that I have ever read. Thanks, guys!"

# Aging
# *Deliberately*

## Paying Attention, Growing, and Thoroughly Enjoying the Ride

STEVE BANNOW AND
TOM SCHNEIDER, MD

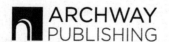

Archway Publishing books may be ordered
through booksellers or by contacting:

Archway Publishing
1663 Liberty Drive
Bloomington, IN 47403
www.archwaypublishing.com
1 (888) 242-5904

ISBN: 978-1-4808-2703-5 (sc)
ISBN: 978-1-4808-2704-2 (e)

Library of Congress Control Number: 2016902901

Print information available on the last page.

Archway Publishing rev. date: 03/15/2016

"I went to the woods because I wished to live deliberately, to front only the essential facts of life, and see if I could not learn what it had to teach, and not, when I came to die, discover that I had not lived."

Henry David Thoreau
From *Walden; or, Life in the Woods*

# *Acknowledgements*

To: Barbara, Bill, Bob, Di, Don, Elissa, Hal, Matt, Mike A, Mike R, Ray, Stewart, Sue, Suzanne, Tom, and Wachinton.

Each of you played a key part in bringing this project to life. Thank you.

With Love,
s

# Preface

Let's start with this: I know people who were old when they were thirty, and I know people who are still young in their eighties and nineties. I'll bet you do, too. I suppose that I have been interested in the aging process in some way or another since I was in my thirties. I really didn't think about what it would be like for *me* to be middle-aged or "elderly," however, until I was in the thick of it—say, about fifty-eight. All of a sudden I began telling others who cared to know my age for some reason that I was "almost sixty." I would make this revelation proudly and hopeful that I might stir up a little surprise. At sixty-four, this practice continues as I often refer to myself as being in my mid-sixties and, again, hope for at least some incredulity on the asker's part. It's a bit egocentric, I suppose, but my approach *is* working. The question then becomes: What exactly is my approach toward aging working *for* or, put another way, what am I attempting to accomplish by making a conscious effort to age deliberately? The answer to this question is not necessarily complicated, but it is extensive and it is important and … it is the underlying theme of this book.

This brings up an interesting question that you very well may be asking yourself: Why does Steve think that *he* has any standing to write a book about aging deliberately? I am so glad that you (may have) asked. My answer is not complicated. I am in very good health—despite a few aches and pains that we will address later—extremely happy, in love, busy with worthwhile activities, and having a jolly good time each and every day of my life. I am also a teacher as well as a life-long student. I like to think that life has taught me a few things that have proven to be helpful as I moved into "middle age" and are proving to be helpful to this very day. I will hasten to add here that lots of what I have learned has been through personal experiences (you know … screw ups[1]) and what I have observed others going through. Consequently, I sincerely believe that I have some ideas to share with you that may either strengthen your resolve to *continue* doing the things that are making the aging process a pleasure and not the enemy or may convince you to consider some changes that just may bring you more joy, fulfillment, and fun as you gain years. I don't expect anyone reading this to feel that it is necessary to embrace and practice every one of my offerings for aging deliberately. *I do* hope, however, that you will at least consider following my lead on at least some of the practices that have brought me a great deal of fulfillment as I have added years to my life.

My point here is that it is up to each of us—working with whatever limitations and gifts we may possess—to make the most of each day of our lives. This means paying attention to balance, trying to make good, healthy, ethical choices regarding our own welfare and that of others, and making the effort to forge ahead … not giving into inertia. In other words, in these pages I am attempting to make my very best case for

---

[1]    Far too much direct exposure to the sun while I was stationed in Hawaii for three years and (fortunately) relatively benign skin cancer on my right temple and chest that followed is just one that comes to mind. I will have more to say about sun exposure in Chapter 7, "Vices."

the practice of aging deliberately—whatever variations to that theme you may choose to make. The rewards, I think you will ultimately agree, are huge—both to you and those around you.

Ultimately, aging deliberately means *growing* as we age, and truly growing as we age takes effort—emotional, intellectual, physical effort. I am convinced that this effort and what results from it makes each day at least slightly better than the wonderful one that preceded it. My hope is that this book will bolster your view if you feel the same way about aging that I do or that it will encourage you to make the effort—and, consequently, find your life more rich and fulfilling—if you currently do not.

— — — — — — — — — — — — — — — — — — — — — — — — —

I would like to make an important point regarding you, our readers. Despite the fact that this book has two sixty-plus-year-old, male authors, we intend it to be written for and to a diverse reading audience consisting of young and older folks, both men and women. Tom and I came to this project after a wide range of experience and study—a huge share of which has been informed by both men and women colleagues, teachers/mentors, friends, family members, and clients and patients of just about every age. We ask that you keep this diverse information base in mind as you make your way through the pages that follow. It is our hope that in doing so you will benefit, as we have, from what others have taught us.

And I have one additional prefatory comment. This one concerns the assembly of this book. It won't take you long to notice that the narrative is not chronological. Tom and I wrote these pages over a period of about a year (October 2014—October 2015)—often writing in the moment when an important thought or event was freshest in our minds. Consequently, you will occasionally read something in one (early) chapter that was actually written well after something that serves as the basis of a key point appearing in a later chapter. The intent was to be immediate and intimate. You, of course, will be the judges of our success in this process.

# *Contents*

# Introduction

We do not *grow* old ....We *become* old
because we *stop* growing.

A s I mentioned in the Preface, I didn't think really seriously about my *own* aging process until my late fifties,
even though I started contemplating it in a more abstract
way more than a couple of decades earlier. Back then, it was
nothing particularly deep or philosophical to me; it was just a
matter of thought, giving the concept some attention. I think
I was also motivated by the fact that I lost my father to a heart
attack when he was only fifty-two after having had two previous MIs at the ages of forty-six and as early as forty. Life is
really good, I thought, and if I want to enjoy it (a lot) longer
than my father did I had better start paying attention. I'll have
much more to say later about how that outlook has charted my
course. For now, let's just say that paying attention to making
intelligent lifestyle choices was not based on the fear of an early
death but on the desire to have a very long, active, full *life*.

More recently, I have been wondering about this: Just
what *is* it like to feel fifty or sixty or seventy or older? I am
not sure that it feels any different to me to be sixty-four than
it did when I was *forty*-four—other than I now run less,

I have no hair on my head to speak of, and I have a lot less stress in my life. I also am in better overall physical condition now than I was then. But just how does it feel to be a certain age past, say, forty? The answer is, I believe, as difficult to articulate as it is to explain a color. (Just how do you explain blue to someone who has never been able to see?) More to the point, I have been told: "Gee, Steve, you certainly don't *look* sixty-four!" That is meant to be a compliment, and I take it as such. But why would someone say that? What does sixty-four *look* like, anyway? Does it mean gray hair? Well, I really don't have any that anyone can see, so maybe that makes me look younger. Does it mean not having lots of wrinkles? Again, I am fortunate and don't have too many of those either. Does it mean not being overweight and actually rather fit? I think we are getting warmer here. And what about attitude and outlook which can often be detected in something unseen, like tone of voice? Yes, I think this is very important. I am fortunate to be a perky guy and you can hear it in my voice. I, for example, have people whom I have never met but have spoken with on the phone tell me that they are quite surprised by my age if the subject comes up: "Gee, you certainly don't *sound* old, Steve." I'll have more to say about this—especially in the next chapter. Now it's time for an anecdote—a real ah-ha moment for me and one that you may be able to relate to.

A couple of years ago, I was in a grocery store in Michigan when I noticed a man who was probably in his early to mid-sixties. He was wearing a T-shirt with writing on the back which was probably meant to be clever or funny, but I didn't think it was either. The back of the shirt featured an overweight, unattractive, very grumpy man who was making a statement:

As I grow older, I just get crabbier.
And I don't care ….
*Deal with it!*


I'm pretty sure that most folks barely noticed the words on the shirt or even the man wearing it, for that matter. Some of those who did may have found what was on the shirt to be mildly amusing while others may have even found something there that they could relate to. For me, the message it sent was anathema. This book is an explication of why I have serious issues with the type of attitude and lifestyle projected by the man who was doubtless older than his years and, I would wager, no longer cared—if he *ever* did.

What struck me at the time I saw the man in the T-shirt—not unlike others I had vaguely noticed previously—was my response to it. Why did it strike me so negatively this time? Why did I—a person whom others regard as funny, quick with a smile and a laugh, and generally able to find humor in just about everything—find the image and the words so utterly unfunny? These are not rhetorical questions, but I am going to leave them unanswered at this time. The answers will unfold in the pages that follow. For now, I will simply say that I, as do many of you, find myself increasingly interested in the aging process—not as something to be feared or loathed but rather as an incredibly complicated and interesting universal something that all of us experience. And, once we move into, say, our forties or fifties, it is helpful, I believe, to realize that the aging process is not the enemy. It can, however, be quite a challenge—one which I have been having a truly wonderful time understanding and undergoing with a certain amount of gusto and, I hope, grace … as well as awe. In other words, I believe that I have been aging *deliberately*.

Let me echo the quotation that serves as the springboard for both this book and my first one[2]—each having the word *Deliberately* so obviously embedded in its title.

> I went to the woods because I wished to live deliberately, to front only the essential facts of life, and see if I could not learn what it had to teach, and not, when I came to die, discover that I had not lived. – H. D. Thoreau

Thoreau's point in these lines is not original. He is getting to something here that others had said—albeit somewhat differently—for centuries previously. He and Confucius and Siddhartha Gautama (the Buddha), Socrates, and others before him and others like Gandhi after him all embrace a profound yet fundamental approach to life. To me it can be boiled down to four words: Pay Attention to Balance. This may seem to be an absurdly simplistic method of understanding what lives behind a truly fulfilling life, but it serves well those who embrace it. Using it to grow and actively engage the aging process rather than to fear or hate it has brought joy to me and to many others. In the chapters that follow, I—along with the help of others who pay attention to balance as well—discuss the things that those of us who wish to garner the benefits of aging deliberately need to pay attention to: what aging actually *is* vis-à-vis fitness, awareness, work, family and friends, spirituality, contemplating death, and more.

I will have plenty to share about the way all of us age, what happens in our bodies that creates the changes that we can see and feel in our physical appearance, thinking and

---

[2] *Traveling Deliberately: Minimizing Stress and Maximizing Fulfillment During Your Journey*

sensing patterns, energy levels, and attitudes. At this point, however, I want to share more with you about how I came to write this book, which I began a week or so after I attended my forty-fifth high school reunion, and why it was so important for me to do so. I suppose the basic concept behind what I have to say has been kicking around inside me for about ten years. It didn't start to take on a real form until I had my first examination by my friend and wellness doc, Tom Schneider. He gave me a really thorough going over: mental acuity tests, an extraordinarily thorough physical checkup, myriad tests of blood, saliva, and other body fluids, and he asked me lots and lots of questions ranging from my average amount of sleep each night to what I ate and when I had my meals to what I did for exercise. When all of the test results were in and Tom had a chance to review the info he had gathered about me and my health, he set me up with a follow-up appointment during which we had a long conversation in his office.

What Tom had to say was very positive. It seems that by eating intelligently, exercising regularly, not smoking, keeping my mind active, and focusing on *Balance* in just about all things in my life I had managed to be and stay very healthy and, to a large extent, keep my increasing number of years to nothing much more than a mere number. You see, it's not that I haven't been paying attention to age. Quite the contrary: I am quite mindful of it and the aging process. But it is this awareness and the resolve to meet the challenges of aging—*deliberately*—that has made and will continue to make all of the difference. Paying attention to the important things in life: love, self-awareness, consideration, personal growth, kindness, balance was, in fact, at the heart of my first book and also consistently informs this one. And, just as I state on several occasions in my *Traveling Deliberately*, I do not profess to have all the answers. I am certain, however, that if you read what I have to say in the pages that follow and give it some thought you may find an approach to doing truly wonderful things during perhaps the most important time of your life as you build your own method of aging deliberately.

As you consider what Tom and I have to say, please focus on the big picture and not the individual pieces of it. What we are offering here is not a formula for a miracle drug which requires that each and every component be added in precise amounts at exactly the correct moment and then processed in a very specific way. Think of this as more of a basic recipe for understanding and actively accepting the process of aging—a recipe with which you should feel free to experiment and flavor to taste. For example, I love to cook but I never prepare the same meal or even a dish exactly the same way that I prepared it before. I am always conscious of using the essential basics—all good stuff—but I do not hesitate to try new things that may push the boundaries a bit. The result is a perpetual parade of wonderful eating experiences that are both fulfilling and delicious. I think that our appreciation of aging and a big-picture-seeing, experimentation-embracing approach to it will help us to enjoy each day of life in very much the same way. Now let's have a look at the first and perhaps most important ingredient—attitude.

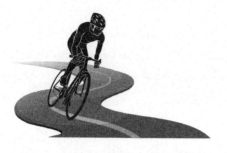

Chapter 1

# Attitude: It All Begins Here

"You are never too old to set another<br>
goal or to dream a new dream."<br>
C.S. Lewis

A quick look at the table of contents of this book and the chapter titles therein will bring to mind a key point: Aging *deliberately* is something that embraces every important component of our existence. While we might have a lively debate about which ones are the most vital, I don't want to get into that here. For me, every chapter contains a rendering of and an approach to aging deliberately that is significant ... and each one needs to be addressed. Every one of us, for our own reasons, may find one or another to be of greater value to our own experience and then tweak a plan for living accordingly. For me, however, the *attitude* that one maintains as one ages is as important an element of the aging process as any—although, for some folks, it is given very little consideration, if any.

Every so often I take a break in whatever I am doing to do an attitude check. I try to be as objective as I can be while I ask myself some questions:

What is my outlook about things in general?

What, if anything, is eating at me?

Who, if anyone (including myself), is bugging me?

What should I be doing about any resident crabbiness, irritation, or downright anger that I may be feeling?

I have gone through this process for years now because I am convinced that harboring irritation, frustration, and resentment (which, after all, are simply other forms of anger) is as antithetical to aging deliberately as drinking a cup of arsenic-laced tea each day.

I will return to the attitude check a little later. For now, however, I want to share some thoughts with you about why our attitudes are so fundamentally important. Let's consider someone we all know: the forty-plus-year-old (we'll call him Larry with my apologies to all of the terrific Larrys out there!) who is fond of saying (often) "I don't *give* a damn what anyone thinks!" Sound familiar? Does this remind you of the T-shirt-wearing guy that I mentioned in my introduction? When Larry says he "… doesn't give a damn …" he is probably referring to just about everything and everyone (including *himself*). This I-don't-give-a-damn attitude is often viewed by the Larrys of the world as a form of ultra-independence or even extreme confidence. In any case, such an outlook is, I believe, based on a really shaky foundation largely composed of ignorance, anger, and fear. You see, it is very likely that Larry has given up … on just about everything. Larry is impatient, quick to think the worst of almost any situation and just about any*one*, in poor physical condition, and probably has hair billowing out of the back of his shirt collar, his nose, and his ears. Some of you may already be thinking I am being unfair if not downright judgmental. Fair enough, but just hear me out. I am not saying that any one thing—especially when it comes to physical appearance—makes someone a Larry. I *am* saying, however, that there are many things—some very obvious and others quite subtle—that reflect our attitudes about life, others, our surroundings, and ourselves.

When I hear a Larry whom I may or may not know say, "I don't give a damn about what anyone thinks…" I usually cringe. Then I find myself thinking, "You know, Larry, life would be a whole lot better for you if you *did*." The thing is Larry just *might* care what *some*one thinks—especially if he has grandchildren—whether he wants to admit it or not. And wouldn't it be great if he could build upon that? In any case, at the heart of the matter is the choice that Larry made at some point to allow himself to become old, and this happened because he chose to stop growing. For whatever reason (e.g., emotional or physical trauma, chronic physical illness, an eating disorder, a vitamin deficiency, financial or personal loss, alcoholism and/or drug addiction, or any combination of these), Larry has allowed the Wonder to leave his life. That said, it is extraordinarily important for me to make a critical point here. I do not include chronic depression in my list of possible "reasons" behind Larry's unfortunate choice. This and certain other mental illnesses go beyond the ability of most people to make the choice to act, to care, and, at some, point to live. This book is not intended to speak to the issues of folks whose illness renders them incapable of making key attitudinal choices without lots of professional counselling and/or medication. For these folks who struggle every minute of every day with issues that most of us can barely relate to—as hard as we may try to do so—I can only offer my most sincere wishes that they (and those who struggle with them) will find peace. Our Larry, however, is not clinically depressed, but he has decided to be angry about aging and to express his anger by giving up the challenge and the Wonder of aging deliberately. The longer Larry remains in this state, the more difficult it will be for him to break out of it by turning to counselling, medication, and/or intense introspection. If he does nothing, he is likely to muddle grudgingly through the rest of his years reacting (often angrily) to one life experience after another.

Now, I will admit that Larry may be an extreme example of the typical PAP (poor-attitude person). Fair enough. I feel certain, however, that virtually any one of Larry's attitudinal characteristics or any combination of those behaviors manifested by his attitude are of concern if left to fester and to become poisonous to a meaningful, rich life. In fact, there is that possibility that Larry may be a lost cause—a person who is perpetually simply unwilling to choose to start living and *aging* deliberately. The good news, however, is that, by far, most of us are not a lost-cause Larry; the ability to make the choice to embrace real, positive changes in attitude is very much within us. The even better news is that most of us only need to make a few key adjustments in our daily activities to see substantial improvement in our lives as we age.

Now let's get back to the attitude check that I brought up

earlier. So how is *your* outlook about things in general? If it is a little less than outstanding, no problem; that, as you well know, is just part of life. Every day is not perfect ... thank goodness! But, if there *is* something really gnawing at you, let's look a little more carefully at what seems to be throwing you off and keeping you preoccupied with too much negativity. What, if anything, is eating at you? Who, if anyone (including yourself) is bugging you? Once you can and do answer those questions, you can go about figuring out what you can do in response.

At the heart of feeling eaten up by something or being really bugged by someone is probably some form of anger. Sure, other strong emotions like sorrow (perhaps over the death of some person or some non-human animal you care about) or disappointment over a missed opportunity, for example, can throw you off your game. But, if you are fairly well balanced and do not succumb to anger at life or others for your setbacks, you will probably start to feel much better in time. What I am driving at is that anger just may be the basis of most of the things that negatively impact our outlooks. Consequently, anger-related issues may influence many of our relationships: with other people, with our work, with our play, with our health, and with everything impacting our lives in general. Ahh, so many possibilities to illustrate this point. Let's consider someone who has lingering but significant anger issues stemming from an ugly divorce that occurred, say, three years ago. We'll call this person Pat—a usefully androgynous name since the scenario I am about to present is something that both men and women can relate to.[3]

---

[3] I use feminine pronouns to refer to Pat to avoid using the awkward he/she, him/her.

Before and during the first twenty years of Pat's twenty-two-year marriage, she was energetic, funny, pleasant, considerate, physically fit, and … fundamentally happy. Pat's spouse's extramarital affair with a younger partner that began at about the twenty-year point in the marriage and which was not well hidden, however, has left her with lots of anger and a fair amount of fear about her future wellbeing and happiness. Pat is full of what-ifs, fundamental questions about self-worth, and sadness. But, most of all, she is consumed with simmering, quiet anger that not too many people can see since she works very hard to hide it. Pat's anger is directed at her ex and the apparently very happy new life that he has with his new partner, at Pat's two children who have decided to remain on good terms with the ex, and, perhaps the worst kind of anger—anger at her Self. Pat's anger's toxins are slowly killing her. She hates her life but, fortunately, she is willing to try to recover. Where to start?

For those of us who have successfully gone through serious anger issues and have come to terms with and eventually overcome them, the answer to the question "Where to start?" is not a surprise. The wonder of it is that it is so very effective. It is also lasting. And, in concept at least, it is quite simple. The answer is tried and true and works in all kinds of anger scenarios. The answer is Forgiveness. Once we accept its importance and its effectiveness, we are able to turn the corner and begin to recover from all the damage caused by the toxic stuff that the anger has created within us. Actually, just about everyone knows that forgiveness is the key, but the really tough part is to come to a point that allows us to forgive—not only the subject of the original anger but also those who have caused secondary anger in us … including ourselves. There is no simple or single prescribed method to accept the concept of forgiveness and put it into play. I suppose religious folks can rely on their faith for the necessary assistance; others may need a more clinical approach with a professional counsellor; others may find the path to forgiveness solely within themselves through meditation and other means; and still others may find any combination of these and other methods helpful. The methods folks choose to use to arrive at the decision that forgiveness is the only real way to take control of their anger is not important. The key is that they ultimately lead to pure, no-strings-attached forgiveness. Once we have learned how to forgive one person, forgiveness of others will follow—with much less difficulty. Free from all the bad feelings that anger and hate foster, the results will likely be the same in virtually every case: a chance for a new and truly fulfilling, meaningful, and fun existence as aging continues—deliberately.

You know, anger is such a devious creature. There are many people past forty or even younger who are just plain angry … and they have no idea why. Other people (especially family members), work, finances, or many other things may have previously brought mostly *pleasant* experiences into the lives of these angry people. But something else is at work here. The fact of the matter is that some folks are angry—*really* angry— about aging itself. They tend to look at it through a retrospective lens, thinking their best years are behind them. This practice is self-deceptive and certainly not helpful. Consequently, it becomes very easy for them to be angry at others—especially younger others—simply because … they are *younger*. Rather than taking positive action to adapt to the aging process and grow with it, they simply become increasingly frustrated with graying hair, aches and pains and stiffness, lost mental acuity, added weight, decreases in hearing and sight, and lost energy and even libido. These angry agers should give forgiveness a try—especially forgiving themselves—but they also need to start making an attempt to push back.

Now, just what *about* this pushing-back business? Well, pushing back is, to a very large extent, much of what this book is about. In addition to paying attention to diet, exercise, work, activity level, awareness, intimacy, appearance, spirituality, and other key ingredients to a full, rich life, sizing up one's attitude and making positive, helpful adjustments to it are extraordinarily effective. And, as I am sure you know, all of these things work together in a hugely important interdependence.

Let me take a little time here to share a couple examples of the types of things that I see virtually every day that touch upon several of the things we have referred to already—specifically anger, aging, and attitude. I am a teacher at heart, by the way, so I find such things helpful when attempting to make a point. More than a few times over the past couple of years I have seen postings on *Facebook* that feature what I call instances of "generational warfare"—anecdotal stories depicting mild to heated confrontations between folks who are Millennials and folks who are Baby Boomers and older. At the heart of these confrontations is the notion that there are fundamental differences between generations ... and the Boomers have it right. They are meant to be clever, amusing, and generationally unifying, I suppose. I find them unfunny, divisive, pretentious, and mean spirited. The theme of the battlefront is this: We are old and wise and you are young and stupid. The most recent example that I saw just the other day described a scenario in which a twenty-something woman who was working at a grocery store checkout counter and mildly chastised a sixty-something shopper who asked for paper bags for her groceries. The point the younger woman was making was that the older woman should have more respect for the planet by bringing her own re-useable bags with her when she shopped for groceries, something the younger generation was far more likely to do. Whether the checkout worker was correct or not in stating her case to the older woman is not the point here. What is essential is to note the tone in the sarcastic and bitter rendition of what happened next as the shopper proceeded to list all the accomplishments of her generation and all of the shortcomings of the "younger generation(s)" followed by a rather nasty bit of name calling. The Boomer and older responses that I see to these sorts of stories are predictable: lots of "likes" and comments in support of the older woman's retort and additional discussion about all that is wrong with "kids" today.

I find nothing positive in the perpetuation of this generational warfare; participating in this one-ups-man-ship is utterly antithetical to the concept of aging deliberately. A little tweaking in attitude on the part of the older shopper could have changed this negative, confrontational battle—with no real winner—into a superb teaching moment. I know, you may be thinking that, as a teacher, I will naturally go to the potential in almost any scenario for a teaching/learning moment. But I am convinced that you don't have to be a teacher by profession to *grow* into one. Just think for a moment what a positive and healthy experience it would have been for both of the folks in my scenario if the shopper had decided to respond with experience, wisdom, and patience to the youthful and perhaps naïve comments of the clerk instead of reacting to them. Certainly some credit needs to be given to the notion of using recycled bags, but that acknowledgement could then lead into a brief history of how the ecology movement really began to take on importance in the sixties and how the shopper used to feel impatience with older folks but found that working together rather than bickering was far more productive.

I could cite many more examples like the one in the previous paragraph, but I want to turn now to a different but related theme: consideration. And I want to begin this part of the discussion by relating something that you might find, at first, to be antithetical to just about everything that I have said so far. What I am about to say has come about not through anger or bitterness or bad experiences as I have aged but rather through *growth*.

Here it is: I am not a subscriber to the Golden Rule as most of us have come to know it. You know what I mean: Do unto others as you would have them do unto you—a principle of ethical reciprocity that is found at the heart of virtually every broadly based world religion and many more local, indigenous ones. My problem with the maxim is not the fact that it extols the notion of behaving in a benevolent way to others; I am very good with that part. Where I break away is the reciprocity component. You see, I sincerely believe that we all should behave in a kind manner to other living creatures—human and non-human animals alike[4]—without the reciprocity piece. In other words: Just do it! Make an effort to be kind, considerate, loving—*period*.

Civility, generosity, patience, consideration should not be practiced on the principle of what-goes-around-comes-around, the Golden Rule, or any other code of ethics or behavior that incorporates reciprocity. Manifestations of kindness should be

---

[4]   I do not necessarily hold this to be an absolute. For example, I find nothing morally or ethically wrong with bumping off small nasty critters that persistently aggressively invade my space and threaten my health. Cockroaches, mosquitos, and tsetse flies come to mind.

part of our lives because they are simply the right things to do. The really cool thing about frequent random acts of kindness is that they just happen to make us feel good about others, about the world in general, and, most important, about ourselves. And this, in turn, does a lot to slow dramatically the negative aspects of aging because the emphasis is on *growth* not anger and *patience* not irritability.

Next, I want to address a more subtle form of attitude/outlook issue that does not seem to be grounded in chronic identifiable anger or hate. Some folks simply become increasingly crabby, inconsiderate, rude, and just plain nasty as they age. We all know some of these individuals for whom being rebarbative seems to them to be an *entitlement*. Their advanced age *entitles* them to be unpleasant. I have seen them act out and they seem to find the grocery shopping experience to be a particularly good spot to express their negativity. It begins with some pretty bad if not aggressive driving to the store followed by taking up two parking spots in the parking lot. Once they get inside the store, there is the habitual leaving their shopping carts in the middle of the aisle while they take forever to make a decision about the bag of chips they want to purchase—only a penny or two separating the virtually identical products.[5] And then there almost always seems to be a need for these folks to berate one of the folks working in the store in a fashion similar to the drubbing they bestowed earlier on the servers at the restaurant where breakfast was eaten an hour before.

I am sure that geriatric medicine specialists and social scientists can offer explanations for the reasons some people

---

[5]  No issues with frugality here—especially for folks on fixed incomes—but much more often than not this penny pinching is more a matter of obstinacy than a need to save.

choose to become a pain in the neck—even when years earlier they were relatively pleasant folks. In fact, for some it is not even so much a matter of making a choice to be a pain in the neck but more a matter of choosing *not* to be pleasant. Perhaps this happens because it might take some extra effort to be positive for a number of age-related issues: an uptick in chronic pain, physical and/or emotional stress brought on by any number of things, disappointment, and/or loss. And this is where virtually all of the rest of this book comes into play. If a person chooses not to give in to the persistent inertia that can accompany aging—and this can take significant effort, especially at first—by finding meaning in the important things in life (work and/or volunteering; involvement with a hobby or community organization; becoming politically, socially, intellectually aware; becoming or staying physically fit; working on one's spiritual side; loving friends, family members, friends, and especially oneself or any combination of these and others) a new, positive, healthy momentum is sure to follow. Nagging crabbiness and crankiness just may give way to patience, consideration, and lots of wonderful reasons to smile.

Just the other day I ran across an article on JAMA (*The Journal of the American Medical Association*) Internet. The lead-in was "People who feel younger at heart live longer." The piece went on to provide scientific evidence to a lot of what I have been driving at in this chapter and what follows in the rest of this book. The authors use the term "self-perceived age" and state that truly believing that you are younger than what your birth certificate says increases your odds for a longer, happier life. Now here is the caveat, and I have alluded to this earlier. Feeling young does not mean acting out like an angry, hormone-ravaged teenager. Being rebellious and obnoxious because an aging person *can* is not manifesting a youthful attitude. The point is that there is nothing wrong with growing *up*; but when we confuse growing up with growing old, problems begin. The JAMA article goes on to provide the example of Fouja Singh who is now 103 and is still running marathons which he began doing about twenty years ago as a means of dealing with his wife's death. Laughter and happiness are central to his life. The authors site him as just one example of folks who choose "…conscientiousness plus optimism…" as their vehicles to consistently make the right healthy, fulfilling choices. I don't think the odds are very good that we would ever see Fouja sporting a crabbiness-themed T-shirt. And, I, for one, will never sport one either.

Other examples of incredibly active, creative, engaged, productive people are all around us. Recently, during a period of just ten days, I was introduced to or reminded of several un-related folks who—despite disabilities, advanced age, personal tragedies—are living wonderfully rich, active lives: Betty (90) from Jackson, Michigan, who does Zumba, line dances, and swims multiple times each week; Ben Vereen, told he would never dance or even sing again after sustaining devastating injuries when he was hit by a car in 1992, is alive and well with a very active *singing and dancing* engagement calendar at age 68; John Kander (composer of *Cabaret, Chicago,* among many others) is still hard at his craft at age 88; Harriette Thompson, a cancer survivor, completed the San Diego Rock n' Roll Marathon (her sixteenth since turning 76) in June 2015 at the age of 92 in less than 7 1/2 hours. In many of such cases, the folks involved did not begin their current notable activities until late in life, proving among other things, that it is *never* too late to get started.

Much of what I have said so far has consistently focused on remaining positive, kind, and considerate. That said, I need to make the following point. I am just as aware as you are that situations and other people will occasionally trigger anger in even the most upbeat person. I do my best not to allow others to control *my* emotional state, but I do have my limits. In other words, I have a temper—just like virtually everybody else. Rudeness, bullying, unchecked greed, prejudice, violence, and a host of other things—whether directed at me or simply occurring nearby—can really get my blood boiling. And, when I sense the need to enter into some unpleasant situation—hackles up, nostrils flaring—I will do so exercising as much control as possible. I believe it is crucial to use one's anger constructively—as a catalyst for a required no-nonsense response to a wrong. The key here is be as balanced and deliberate as we can be, never taking things any farther than is absolutely necessary—a stepped approach. I remain vigilant with my boundaries and I know that some things are just not within my skill set to handle. Sometimes reinforcements (e.g., police or others better trained and/or equipped to handle specific types of potentially violent situations) may be absolutely necessary. The point is that I don't try to completely repress my anger when it is summoned by circumstances. After all, it is a natural and often healthy response to certain things. What I *do* try to do is to keep to a minimum those situations that cause me to become angry, to direct or channel my anger in a positive direction, and to let go of it as soon as I can.[6]

---

[6] One of the greatest proponents of channeling anger into positive results was one of my all-time heroes, Jackie Robinson. As anyone who is an athlete knows, there are very few things that can be done well in sports when one is angry, but Jackie had the unique ability to use his anger in a positive way—on and off the field. And when he was on the field he was almost always angry and he was always really, really good.

I once read somewhere that a good way to deal with bad conduct is not to condemn the person who commits it but to condemn only the *behavior* and to work on *teaching* the person. This is noble advice and I strive to embrace it although part of me succumbs, more often than I like, to reactionary anger when I am confronted with cruelty, harmful greed, racism, hatred, and/or other despicable behavior. I like the concept of focusing on the behavior, not the person, because it balks at condemning other people as a general practice. And I think it is an excellent principle to live by when dealing with children or others who are still *open* to advice and/or instruction. As I have added years to my life, I do tend to give just about anyone the benefit of the doubt in this regard. That said, I am still working on dealing with channeling my very negative feelings when contemplating the likes of a Bernie Madoff, or a Dick Chaney, or a Fred Phelps (now deceased former pastor of the Westboro Baptist Church) or … or any number of people who whose actions I perceive to be utterly deplorable. I think the answer may lie somewhere in the process of giving such things real attention and thought in the first place and doing our very best to exercise patience and forbearance first before resorting to judgment and condemnation. I pay attention to things and, consequently, see *lots* of bad stuff. So, I will probably be working on this very challenging goal for many years to come.

As you reflect on what you have read so far and consider what the subjects of the next sixteen chapters deal with, try to keep in mind how significant each one is—not only in its own right but also with respect to the others and what a huge part attitude has to play in these relationships. Once these components are in *Balance*, aging deliberately becomes natural, fun, and very healthy.

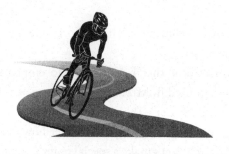

Chapter 2

# Limitations and Rising Above the Natural Forces of Gravity[7]

Please consider the central theme of the extraordinarily profound yet highly practical "Serenity Prayer" attributed to Reinhold Niebuhr. It is, of course, an appeal to a higher power to grant the requestor the ability to accept those things in life that cannot be changed and the wherewithal to change the things that can and should be changed and, perhaps most important, the insight to grasp the difference between the two. I encourage you to find a copy of it in its entirety, to read it, and to reflect upon it—often. For understandable reasons, the "Serenity Prayer" has been relied upon and made part of the basic working tenants of a number of

---

[7] Please see Appendix I for a story from my adolescence that may be helpful here.

organizations, including, perhaps most notably, Alcoholics Anonymous.

The three ideas that I would like to emphasize in this chapter are captured in Mr. Niebuhr's prayer: acceptance, action, and introspection. These relate to everything in life, of course, but here we are going to consider how they relate to aging deliberately. Let's make a special point to remember—as we move on to other topics after this chapter and reflect on those that preceded this one—what we consider in depth here. I will remind you.

So, let's consider what we cannot change. Interestingly, I don't think we can even start to name such things until the third component of the prayer comes into play. I am referring to knowing the difference between what each of us can (and should) change and what each of us cannot change, that is to say *introspection*. My point is that some things cannot be changed by anyone: the distance between the earth and the moon. Some things can be changed by some folks but not others: what Ted Turner decides to do with the millions of acres of land that he controls. But I think this point is best used if we take it personally, close to home. If each of us were to make a list, some things would be different and many would overlap. Most important, I think, is change vis-à-vis others who are close to us. I cannot make one of my best friends go to a pool and swim for half an hour three times a week and I cannot make her like classical music as much as I do. Please keep these things in mind as we move along.

Now, have you ever noticed how folks—often with a smile and a wink—attribute the body bagging and sagging that accompany old age to "gravity?" This seems to me to be a good natured yet passive way of acknowledging and also giving in to some of the effects of the aging process. Fair enough … for *now*. More on pushing back against bagging and sagging later. The reality is that, for many of us who really have made the most of our lives, the years have brought more than wonderful experiences. Participating in sports, having accidents, feeling the effects of some of the unpleasant genetic gifts of our parents (some of which are with us from birth), having and rearing children, and many other components of existing for more than a few decades do take their toll. In a word, they present us—*each* of us—with *limitations*.

In Chapter 1, I focused on the importance of attitude—maintaining a *positive* attitude—as we age deliberately. I was not doing so because I think being positive comes easily every moment of every day. It doesn't … not for me and not for you. It takes effort. In the spirit of full disclosure, let me share some of the things that challenge my choice to remain positive. My purpose in sharing some of my more significant potential limitations is to assure you that you are not alone with yours and to be clear about the fact that there really are ways to deal positively and constructively with lots of things that come into play as we age.

Let's talk about pain—physical, constant, chronic arthritic pain. I have it. In fact, most of the reason that I have a fifty percent disability from the military is directly related to osteoarthritis. I am not sure *why* or *how* it started at about the age of thirty-five and has consistently spread throughout my body—pretty much head to toe. It certainly was not an issue for either one of my parents. In fact, my father played college football and professional baseball and was even banged up rather severely during WWII and never seemed to have any arthritis issues. Perhaps he didn't live long enough to manifest any symptoms. He died from a heart attack—his third—at the age of fifty-two. I will have much more to say about *his* health issues and how they influenced my lifestyle choices later in the book. I stopped wondering why I was arthritic about fifteen years ago when I realized that I needed to do more than simply accept my condition passively. And here is where the wisdom of the "Serenity Prayer" comes into play. I found that I really *can* accept the limitations of my arthritis (e.g., no more running—a lifelong love), but that doesn't mean I have to give up. You see, the arthritis, for me, is a condition and, yes, a limitation; it is *not* a life sentence to passivity. I deal with it by pushing back, by *moving*—as much as I can in ways that may be painful but will not damage me. Many of you are familiar with the expression that certain activities may hurt but the hurting is "good" soreness/pain. That's what I am referring to.

My life is a blur. I am in almost constant motion just as I was during my Navy career and even as an adjunct English prof and as a community college department head and dean. I move. And it is this movement—along with channeling/meditation—that, even though it causes me lots of "good" soreness, allows me to keep going—without pain pills. I suppose I am fortunate to be a naturally high-strung and perky guy—not considered by my elementary teachers to be a particularly attractive feature—but I also have made the choice to stay active and, consequently, to dramatically improve my chances of a long, healthy, rewarding life. Sure, no more running for me, but now I ride my bicycle, walk, swim, canoe with Barbara, kayak, lift weights, and do a whole lot of other stuff that I did not do when I was running. Despite my arthritis limitation, I am as fit as I have ever been and my body fat is less than nine percent. My chapters on fitness and eating/drinking go into far more detail on such things, but right now I need to share some more of my health issues that could be considered to be limitations.

Now let's consider something many of us deal with—or don't: hypertension; you know … high blood pressure. Yes, I have it, as I am certain my father did. So, let's talk for a bit about what health strengths and challenges our parents pass along to us. I will focus on the Old Man for a minute. (George is his name, and we will be referring to him later on as well.) See if this resonates with you or one of your parents. My father played football at the University of Illinois and professional baseball. He was also a WWII hero although it took others to let me know that. George was a handsome, vital, toned, vain, and charismatic guy. He was also a three-pack-a-day cigarette smoker until his first heart attack at the age of forty on New Year's Day, 1962. He was able to kick the habit but his heart had been seriously damaged. He also continued to live with lots of business-related stress, drank too much, and was ignorant—through no real fault of his own, considering the virtually unknown state of preventive medicine in his day—of what he needed to do to keep himself really healthy. He had a second heart attack in 1967 and a third, which killed him, in 1973—about a month after his fifty-second birthday. I am letting you in on this because I learned from his mistakes and I have outlived him because I know and practice what health practices he didn't. It would not be overstating the case to say that in dying young and really getting my attention in doing so, he has given me life—healthy, fulfilling Life.

So…back to hypertension. The good news is that I know that I have it; there are some things that I can do about it; and I do those things—religiously. So, what is it that I do to push back against hypertension? First, I take my meds (Hydrochlorothiazide and Losartan Potassium). I know that, for some folks, changes in diet and exercise alone can be the answer to controlling high blood pressure. Believe me; I have tried lots of combinations to do this naturally—to no avail. I need to take my meds. And … they, along with my diet, exercise regime, and stress control, have been working very well, indeed. I know because I check my blood pressure almost every morning. Second … well, I just mentioned it: a combination of a reasonable, essentially healthy diet, an intelligent, consistent exercise program, and limiting stress (through meditation and the other things that I have already mentioned). You can see how everything seems to be integrated. And it works!

And what about high (bad) cholesterol? Yes, a higher than healthy amount of it occurs naturally in me. Again, exercise, diet, and meds have turned this into a non-issue for me.[8] I first discovered that my cholesterol was "naturally" high (consistently in the mid to high 140s with very low good cholesterol/HDLs) in the late 1980s. After trying just about everything I could do to lower it through diet and exercise, I discovered Simvastatin in 2003. With exercise, a healthy diet, and this amazing drug, my cholesterol is text-book good these days and, knock on wood, no side effects like increased liver numbers to report.

There is much more that I could tell you about various things that have been limitations for me for a long time and others that are relatively recent issues in my life. The point is that we all have them. The important question becomes: What are we going to do about them? My experiences with golf and running may strike a chord with you.

---

[8]  Tom and I will have lots more to say about diet, exercise, meds, and supplements later in the book.

I started playing golf when I was about eight. I played a long time—decades—before I started playing consistently well. My friends used to say "Steve has always wanted to play golf very badly … And he does." After years of struggle and frustration, I finally found a teaching pro who could help me. He started by teaching me the real mechanics of the game— the physics behind what happens when a golf club strikes a golf ball and what needs to be done to be consistently successful at doing so. He then broke my swing down completely and even experimented with having me play left-handed. After about two months of instruction and playing lessons, I really started to get it. My improvement was impressive to say the least and by the end of that season I was playing to about an eight handicap. I was forty-two and happy to say that you really *can* teach old(er) dogs new tricks!

However, there was a dark cloud growing over my progress on the golf course. It had begun to form a few years before my significant improvement. It was arthritis—especially in my lower back. If you are a golfer, you probably know what is coming. When you play golf (and eschew riding around in a golf cart), you are either standing or swinging a club—the two things that, by far, caused me the greatest discomfort. The arthritis worsened over the next several years, and it became increasingly difficult for me to play golf. It was as if I only had so many swings in me each week. And this meant I could play about once a week with virtually no practice without experiencing really serious pain. I did not, however, throw in the towel—at first. I went to pain specialists for treatments, consistently performed all of the appropriate stretching exercises, and saw chiropractors for adjustments. Nothing was working to relieve the increasing pain. Not being able to practice and only able to play about eighteen holes a week, it will come as no surprise that my game really started to deteriorate. I was in for some big changes.

In 1997, I received orders to transfer to Hawaii to be the Officer in Charge of the Navy Legal Service Office Detachment at Pearl Harbor. Hawaii is truly a golfer's paradise, but it was not to be one for me. About three weeks before I was to leave for Hawaii, I was playing golf with my usual group. I was in serious pain but I was playing unusually well over the first six holes. In fact, I was one under par when I hit my approach shot within about six inches of the cup on the seventh hole. My second birdie of the round was a virtual certainty. As I walked up to the green, it hit me: I was finished. I told my golf buddies that I was done and would meet them at the clubhouse. They were dumbfounded. I was quitting while having a great round and didn't even knock in the birdie putt. I had an early lunch and a couple of beers, did a little reading, and watched a sports show as I waited for my friends. I also did plenty of thinking about my decision on the course. I was quite happy with it.

When my friends joined me a couple of hours later, they were still astonished by my decision to walk away from such a great round—even though they were well aware that I had been dealing with significant pain while playing golf for quite a while. I explained that I was not only done playing for the day, but I was, in fact, done playing golf ... for *life*. I explained that the pain was just too much and I was not having fun anymore. There were plenty of protests and calls for more medical steps to be taken, but my resolve was obvious. I was done. I recognized my limitation; I was OK with it; and I was ready for something new. That something new turned out to be an entirely new pastime—SCUBA diving, something I had always had an interest in but had never tried. And, after all, I was going to Hawaii.

Within a couple of weeks after landing in Honolulu, I was taking SCUBA lessons. I became a skilled diver and never looked back (to golf)—not once! So the point of all this is adaptation. Once it became clear to me that my golf game was deteriorating as my arthritis intensified, and there was virtually nothing that reasonably could be done to remedy the situation, I decided to make some changes. I did not become depressed or bitter about my situation; I simply faced facts, found something new to keep me active and interested, and went ahead with life. I had experienced a major limitation but used it as a springboard to become involved in something new and exciting. I don't know if I would have ever learned to dive if I had not turned away from golf.

Unlike golf, my running came easily. I was always fast. My speed was a great asset in virtually every sport I was involved in. (I can't say it was much help in golf!) I was a sprinter and a long jumper in high school and college. Later, in my thirties, I became involved in distance running and loved it. Running was a great way to burn calories, release stress, stay in decent physical condition, and be alone with my thoughts. Running became more than a hobby or an exercise routine. For me, as is the case for many runners, it became an integral part of my life. I did not run with others unless I was in a race and I never used an I-Pod or more antiquated music-administering gadgets. I preferred the sounds of my own breathing and footsteps, nature, and the occasional aggressive dog's ambush noises.

While I enjoyed golf and tennis (which I also had to give up), as well as the social side of the games, I was in love with running. For about twenty years both golf and running were key components of my life; they helped to identify me. Additionally, my involvement with each became increasingly limited as wear and tear and arthritis continued to take their toll. Running in pain was a given for me, but once the endorphins kicked in things were at least tolerable. The main issue for me was that my knees were becoming so battered that I was doing serious structural damage to them and was sustaining injuries requiring surgery by doing nothing other than running. By 2006, the baker's cyst behind my right knee had become so large that I could not bend my knee backward more than about seventy-five percent of the way. It was clear that my running days had to end. I can't say that I was completely devastated because I had sensed the end was coming for a year or more. That said, I was very sad to say good-bye. Running—from racing around the neighborhood as a little boy to competition in track and field as a young man to distance running as an adult—had been a part of my life for as long as I could remember. Facing yet another limitation—this one especially significant—I had to decide what I would do in response: throw in the towel on exercise or find something else. Throwing in the towel meant giving up, ceasing to grow, and allowing gravity to win.

I tried something else. I started to incorporate a wide variety of physical activities into my life. Rather than depending on running and an occasional round of golf or tennis game to keep me physically active, I took on all kinds of activities that were much more back and knee friendly. At first, it was cycling, walking, and a mat workout a couple of times a week. But I continued to add things: kayaking, canoeing, stationary rowing, stationary cycling, elliptical, chin-ups, resistance training, abdominal conditioning, and much more focused core work. (I did give yoga a valiant effort, but I found that I left my sessions far more sore and stressed than I was when I walked in.) After a few months, I was able to let go of running completely and to embrace this new, much more diverse fitness program. I started to feel even better than I did when I was running as I was now working on every part of my body. And now that I have been at this new regime for about eight years, I can say that I am in better overall physical condition at sixty-four than I was at thirty-five! I had discovered something really important about fitness as I transitioned from a program that was based almost exclusively on running to a varied approach. I think that I can hear some of you saying the magic word right now: *balance.*

Now, it's time for Doc Schneider's take.

Ahh, limitations, thanks for bringing *that* subject up, Steve! And, while I'm at it, thanks for allowing me to introduce myself by rendering a list of my own. Seriously, I am glad Steve took this approach. Having a chance to share, at the outset, some of my own health and life-style challenges is actually a really good way to get started. It is important to be keenly aware of our limitations—not to be lessened by them but, instead, to be motivated by them. Also, by knowing more about me and my limitations, you may be able to get a better grasp on why I do what I do in both my personal and professional lives and how it all ties up into my own take on aging deliberately.

Firstly, I am in my 71$^{st}$ year, not including uterus time. My careers have been multiple but three biggies have hindered my health. The first was as a fighter pilot in Vietnam. Evidently, I wasn't that good of a pilot because I was shot down twice and landed in Agent Orange. (Turns out Agent Orange is not a sunscreen after all.) My second career was as a physician/surgeon. I've since learned that such a career path is peppered with stress, to state in mildly. And my third "career" in my younger years—mostly during the days that I was involved in careers one and two—was as a body abuser. This was done, to a large extent, with the help of the Marlboro man and Jack Daniels. Now, I'm not admitting to mere dabbling, mind you. Oh no! I'm talking about world class, Olympic-level consumption. In later years, my doc would ask me how much I smoked, and I would reply that it would be easier to calculate how much I breathed. Did I mention food? My weight hit 294! (Now it is 185). And along with the scenarios I just depicted came the following: diabetes, renal failure, cancer, hypertension, high lipids (fats), gout, arthritis, coronary artery disease, bypass surgery, five coronary stints, sepsis (infection throughout the body) resulting in a four-month stretch in the ICU, neuropathy, hepatitis, malaria, perforated small intestines, obesity, COPD (bad lungs), abdominal abscesses (six) .... And now I think I am about to have an ingrown toenail! So, seriously, the Agent Orange and a truly lousy lifestyle definitely put me in the hurt locker with each of the above episodes. The fact that I have learned from all that I have gone through is the reason I am here today. Much of what I have learned informs all that I will be saying within this book. Nice to be with you!

I think it is pretty clear that Tom has had more than his fair share of health difficulties that have created their own unique SchneiderWorld realm of limitations. Yet, through it all, he has found a way to stay focused, as well as he can possibly be, positive, and—most important—fundamentally happy. He asked that I share his GAGE principle with you here. I think it works quite well with what we discussed about attitude and outlook in Chapter 1, as well.

In my practice, patients have come to me for a wide variety of complaints, but each one wanted one thing: To be happy. They may have thought happiness would come from fewer wrinkles, more muscles, a magic pill, or a sudden bonanza of big bucks. But, of course, that sort of thing never works. In fact, some of saddest and most depressed people today are winners of the lottery. So what's the answer? Well, I'm surely not the guru of giddiness. But I have found a simple formula to remind me of how to stay focused on happiness—despite our limitations. The mnemonic is GAGE.

*The G is for gratitude.* I take a deep breath and am thankful for that simple act of breathing. There was a time when a respirator had to do that for me and I "watched" as my lungs filled and then emptied—the sound of the machine reminding all of us in the room of the seriousness of my condition. I never take a breath for granted.

*The A is for acceptance.* Gotta tell ya; this is a tough one for me. I'm still working on it. It reminds me that whatever comes my way will pass. Even the good times, but especially the bad ones. Tough for me to remember when I've just been cut off on the highway with my daughter in the car. I feel the rage rising within me like a wind storm. Chillax, Tom. That guy is on his way to his own funeral ... but not with me! Yes, I know I should be less judgmental and of a gentler heart. But, like I said, I'm still working on this one.

*The second G is for generosity.* Now this one is just plain fun! Giving to others is such a kick. Yes, we should give to our family and friends, of course, but I'm talking about giving to the invisible people in our lives, as well: the checkout clerk, the waiter, the person walking by you on the street, the barber, the gal at the coffee shop, and thousands more whom we seldom really see in our lives. Let's work on giving them a smile for the day. Let's get away from the standard lines like "fine" when asked "How are you doing?" Why not try something else? "Better for seeing you!" would do nicely. Good bye could become "Hope your day is fast and fun." Anything that you say that is positive and different from the norm will tell people that you care. Yes, even when you don't! Because this is all about selfish giving. The more you give, the better you get to feel. So help me, it's the truth. I remember buying my wife some flowers at the grocery store and the elderly cashier noted how pretty they were and asked "who are they for?" "They're for you, of course," I said. I swear as I write this, she started to cry. As you can imagine, my wife smiled broadly when I told her why there were no flowers for her that day. Now, I know in my heart that I'm not always that good of a guy, but, on days like that, I think I am.

And now the E. What the heck does that stand for? It's the answer, of course. GAG=E. *E is for enjoyment.* And that's exactly what you get when you add GAG to your day. It's the best formula that I have found to keep me relatively sane day to day—although my wife claims that even though I may be "enjoying," I am light years from sane!

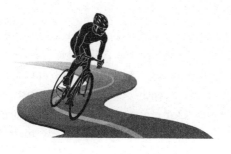

Chapter 3

*Inflammation and the Science of Aging: Inflammation Sinflammation!*

Y ou have already heard from my friend and co-conspirator in this project, Dr. Tom Schneider—also known to those who know and love him as Uncle Tommy, Doctor Tom, Doc, Earth Man, Dad, Daddy, Gramps, and, well, you get the idea. You are going to hear a lot more from him in some of the chapters that follow, but considering all the really good stuff he has to say, nothing is more important to your excellent overall health and longevity—the subject of this book—than his comments in this chapter. But first, it is high time for some background info on my friend.

Tom and I first met while we were in the Navy during a brief doctor-patient encounter in Newport, Rhode Island, where we were both stationed in late 1983. Our paths crossed again about eight years ago. Both of us had retired from the Navy and I was head of the Allied Health Department at Pensacola Junior College. A group of us from the college had come to visit the recently-opened Andrew Institute in Gulf Breeze, Florida. Our group was assembled in the conference room for an opening briefing with a few members of the Andrews staff when Tom, who was in charge of the Institute's Wellness Center at the time, walked in—joking, relaxed, and pleasant. He had mischief in his eye and I liked him (as did all of us visitors) instantly. Tom and I started to rib each other—openly—almost immediately. Soon thereafter, he was my wellness doc and very soon after that we were friends for life.

Tom Schneider has been around the block a few times—and then some. Originally from Carlisle, Pennsylvania, where he was born at the Army War College Campus, he did his undergraduate work at the College of the Holy Cross (Bachelor's degree, Classics and Classical Languages, 1967) and at Columbia University, Iona College, and Manhattanville College (Bachelor's degree, Premed, 1973). He received his medical degree from the Georgetown University School of Medicine (Family Practice, Facial Plastics, Bariatrics, ENT, Ethics, and Pain Management) in 1977. His internship and residencies over thirty-plus years could fill a page or two. From January 1964-September 1989, Tom was on active duty in the US Navy completing two separate careers as a fighter pilot and as a physician. He retired as an O-6 (Captain). He is also a truly gifted teacher, an athlete, a scholar, a husband, a father, a grandfather, and a fantastic friend. He is currently the Director of *Healthspan* based in Pensacola, Florida, and has focused his practice on Preventative Medicine since June 2000. Tom has authored numerous publications, perhaps the most provocative of which is *A Physician's Apology: Are We Making You Sick?* (Indigo River Publishing, 2013). He is an outspoken advocate for fitness and preventative medicine and an avid rower (especially when in the company of his young daughter, Ellie).

Years before I even thought about writing this book. I had my first Schneider exam. It was, by far, the most in-depth physical examination/evaluation I have ever received—blood tests, saliva tests, urine samples; you name it. And questions, lots and lots of questions. Once all of the data was in, Tom brought me back in for a thorough briefing on his findings. I am delighted to say that, had my physical examination/evaluation been a college exam, I would have aced it. Seems like I had been doing a lot of things—diet, exercise, sleep, dealing with stress—really well. I just did not fully understand why what I was doing was working so well. Tom explained why … and gave me lots and lots of extremely important info for really good health maintenance. You see his goal was and very much still is not to treat his patients *after* they get sick. His objective is to help us stay fit, happy, and well so that acute, reactive medical treatment is, for the most part, unnecessary. Tom is really smart, very funny, deeply committed to his profession, and passionate in his caring—about just about everyone. He also knows a whole lot about aging and the key contributors to good health as well as those things that are serious threats to staying well—particularly as the years add up. There are a number of things I could have asked him to write about at this point[9], but I concluded that

---

[9] One of the more fascinating areas of research regarding the aging process deals with telomeres—an essential component of human cells that have a direct impact on how our cells age. They may also be tied directly into the onset and advancement of cancer. I admit to having very limited knowledge about telomeres, but I am learning. I am particularly interested in the work of Dr. Al Sears, MD, and Nobel Laureate, Dr. Elizabeth Blackburn, PhD. I intend to do much more research in this remarkably compelling area of science, and I urge you to do the same. Perhaps we can get together and share our notes some day!

a discussion of the very important but often misunderstood role that inflammation plays in our lives was probably the most useful. Fortunately for all of us, Tom was willing to take this on.

Take it away, Tom....

I remember it clearly. The day was one of my best. My daughter and wife were out shopping and, yes, my feet were up as I read one of my favorites. Ahh, peace. God was in his heaven and all was right with the world and then I heard it. The words and melody to "Sitting on the Dock of the Bay" by Otis Redding came smoothly from my cell phone. Peace no more. But wait, the name of the caller flashed "Steve" and I was once again back to "all's right with the world." Why? Because the only "Steve" in my phone is the one and only "King of the Road" and long-standing friend, Steve Bannow. This was truly a treat. And in no time we had caught up with each other's lives and I was lustfully listening to Steve's latest travels and adventures. I'd be lying if I told you that I wasn't a bit jealous of Steve and his wanderlust, but please don't feel bad for me. After all, every night I have the joy of fractions, decimals, and spelling words to review with my ten-year old Ellie. I bet Steve doesn't know that "gray" can also be spelled with an "e" and it means exactly the same thing. Take that, Steve!

It didn't take Steve long to ask a favor of me. My first guess was that he'd run out of protein powder and would I be kind enough to forward him the latest and greatest. But no; his request was, indeed, much more flattering. Would I kindly contribute a few words to his new book? Not a nanosecond passed before I jumped like a fly to a Venus fly trap. What a treat! But the other shoe hadn't fallen yet.

"Fantastic, Steve, and of course I'd be delighted," I said naively. "What's the topic?" I was really hoping it wouldn't be a toughie like "World Peace" or "The Meaning of Life."

"No, no Tom. I'm looking for a summary on inflammation."

"Excuse me? Inflammation? Could I please have 'World Peace' and 'The Meaning of Life' instead?"

Now don't get me wrong. Inflammation is actually one of my favorite topics, but it is amazingly complex and encompassing. Two or three volumes and maybe we can hit the highlights. But a chapter....Yikes!

When we hear the word, inflammation, most of us think of an evil dragon salivating to bring us down. Not a single good thing can be said about that villain. But I'm here to defend my ol' buddy, inflammation. So let's start with its meaning. As usual, it comes from the Latin, *inflammatio*, meaning to fire up. But we all know what it is. Who hasn't scraped a knee, or had a bee sting? That's when we see it: redness, swelling, and pain.

Now what about that makes it my "buddy?" Well here's the thing. If you get a splinter under your skin, you'll get those same telltale signs of inflammation. And in this and every case of inflammation, it is your body's response to injury. You have a built in immune system that goes into battle station mode to wall off an abscess, splinter, cut, ingrown hair...anything that's attacking your homeostasis (big word meaning normal state of health). An absolutely miraculous fire department for your body. So you can see that inflammation is our lifesaver. In fact, without it, we wouldn't live a day. Inflammation: so often maligned and yet so critical for our well-being.

So we now know that splinters, insect bites, allergies, and a ton of other everyday warriors attack us. And their attacks enable our defense protectors to move into action and keep us healthy. A simple way of looking at a truly complex system in our body (our immune defenses) is to know that it kicks into gear when we smoke, exercise, drink alcohol, stress out, not sleep, eat lots of sugar, get angry, and …well, you get the point. (And, by the way, we do those things when we're stressed or depressed). We have a "feel good" brain hormone (neurotransmitter) called serotonin that makes us feel good. Now what do you think raises serotonin? Yup, smoking, Cinnabon sugar rolls, wine, exercise, and all the goodies in life. So get a little down, get a tad panicky, like when you are trying to get through the TSA gauntlet at an airport when you're late for a flight (Whew, made it with a few minutes to spare!) and there you have it: stress! Now, look around for a broccoli bar. Nope. But there are plenty of Cinnabons, chocolate chips, and soft pretzels around to be washed down with a super mocha breve latte with extra whipped cream. Ahh! Now I'm ready for the packed plane with leg crunching seats and the guy in front of me that just has to have his seat recline on my knee caps because of the extra ten degrees of reclining that will make his flight so much the better! Stress and anger. (I sure hope they have a Coke and one of those ginger cookies ready for me after we reach altitude!)

What did we just do? Well chemically, we created little critters called "free radicals." These little fellows attack us. And good old sugar hooks up with the protein in our blood (called glycation) and that marriage is like a bowling ball with spikes on it. Imagine how pleasant that is as it rolls down your arteries causing … yup, you've got it: inflammation.

Here's an interesting tidbit. That inflamed artery lining is now like a scraped knee that you gave yourself as a child learning to ride a bike. Your body responded by covering it with a scab to protect it from infection. Wouldn't it be great if we had a similar system internally? Well, we do. Remember that horrific stuff called cholesterol? A name worse than ISIS. But guess what? We make cholesterol in our liver and it makes most of our hormones like testosterone, progesterone, estrogen, and cortisol. Yup, it's a critical substance for keeping us alive. Unlike the current advertisements try to suggest, it is not meant for selling statins (cholesterol lowering medicines). Now here's the tidbit as promised. Chole means liver. Sterol is like a steroid (used for taking down inflammation). Thus, cholesterol is a substance made in the liver that produces hormones and lowers inflammation. Now where was our last deposit of inflammation? Oh yeah, on our artery walls. Cholesterol and a host of other anti-inflammatories cover the artery inflammation. So lo and behold, cholesterol is not a problem. It's the free radicals and glycation that are the real culprits.

You may be thinking that there's not much difference in our friendly protective inflammatory response to a bee sting than there is in the same protective inflammatory action on our arteries. Well, there really are some big differences. It's like the difference between a 5K run (being short of breath, hot, and sweaty) and a marathon (being exhausted). But the next day after the marathon, every muscle aches, your mind is not quite firing on all cylinders, and you are fatigued for a number of days.

Inflammation has a 5K component (acute). That bee sting is red, sore, and swollen but clears with our immune system shortly. And you feel the symptoms right away. The marathon inflammation (chronic) from smoking is a sly fox. We don't feel the damage for years. Every puff is beating up our arteries, throwing free radicals at our lungs, and sending them to our brain as well. Just like consuming tons of processed sugar. We don't feel or sense the inflammation acutely but the damage is relentless.

And by the time we do notice the symptoms, the proverbial horse is long gone out of the barn. We have heart disease, shortness of breath, cancer, pain, dementia, and possibly many more serious health concerns. Unfortunately, most of these diseases and symptoms are irreversible. Why didn't we see this coming? There are a couple of big reasons. First, chronic inflammation is a silent killer. And second, the causative habits tend to temporarily make us feel better. Remember good old serotonin? Sugar, nicotine, alcohol, etc. make us feel good, and thus, we keep indulging. Who doesn't want to feel good?

How do we possibly overcome this dilemma? Well, this is both very easy and very hard. It doesn't take a *Jeopardy* show winner to figure out that we need to find an alternative to Cinnabons, Twinkies, or … the forbidden fruit of your choice. Easy peasy! Really? I think not. Changing and saying "No, not now" to our feel good is so much easier said than done. But notice please that I said, "No NOT NOW." I didn't say simply "NO." 'Cause let's face it. For most of us, "No" just won't make it … at least not for long. For example, I'm diabetic and use insulin. Can I ever have a 31 Flavors Jamocha ice cream again? You bet I can. But why? Because it tastes so darn good! Now here's the kicker. I have it once a month and I get the child's cup. I love every lick. But I don't have it every day or every week. Too many spiked bowling balls and free radicals for my kidneys, brain, and heart.

I'm pretty sure that someone a whole lot smarter than I am (Socrates, I think) said: "Everything in moderation." And so it is today. We must learn to stop fighting ourselves with inner voices saying, "Yes I can; no I can't." I remember when I was hooked on the deadly tobacco plant. What I wouldn't do for a Marlboro after coffee in the morning. When my son was born, I just had to try giving them up. Secondhand smoke is just as deadly and horrendous for children. Try as I might though, I kept opening a new pack. I used pills and a dial-down ciga-rette holder and, yes, I even went to menthols. I kept fighting myself: "Stop you wimp! Do it for your kids! But I desire some pleasure. But my dad smokes and he's seventy-five. But ..." Well, you get the picture. In fact you've probably painted your own picture by now.

And then a patient of mine, who was a psychiatrist, mentioned the tobacco smell on me and asked if I'd like to quit. Skeptical, I agreed and he took me through a course in self-hypnosis. Interestingly, my mantra while doing self-hyp-nosis was not against smoking. It went something like this: "Smoking [insert your own Achilles heel] tastes great. I like smoking. It makes me feel good. I CAN smoke. But don't need to hurt myself or my family any more. I CHOOSE not to smoke right now." I haven't smoked in forty years. Whenever I had the urge, I would just self-hypnose. Eventually, I replaced daily self-hypnosis with daily exercise. I chose rowing and now sport calluses on my hands. Calluses versus lung disease and atherosclerosis. I'll take the calluses.

So now we have two forms of inflammation: acute and

chronic. We really want our immune system up and running full bore to help fight illnesses and infections. Interestingly, most, not all, chronic inflammation conditions are brought into our systems by our own doing. And yes, there are genetic proponents of our individual make up that make us more susceptible to certain diseases. But regardless of the name applied (cancer, multiple sclerosis arthritis, fibromyalgia, ulcer … etc.), the underlying cause is always inflammation.

How about you? Do you have active chronic inflammation right now? Remember, you seldom feel the symptoms until the disease is fully present. For example, just about all adults have periodontal disease. Bacteria reside under the gum line See, your hygienist was right. Floss, floss, and floss some more … those bacteria under the gum line are right next to your blood vessels and can emit inflammatory proteins to every part of your body. They elevate sugars in diabetes, exacerbate joint pain in arthritis, and even affect closure of coronary vessels on the heart. Interestingly, my doctor has never told me to see a dentist! So let's assume you have some inflammation. How can we tell? Well nowadays there are labs that can help. Although seldom ordered routinely, your physician can order a homocysteine level and a C-Reactive Protein (CRP) test. These are readily available and can give a clear marker for your inflammation and the degree of it. As inflammation becomes more understood, more and more labels will be available. For example, hs-CRP (or high-sensitivity/heart specific C-Reactive Protein) can be used to localize inflammation in the heart and artery linings.

"So what?" you may be wisely asking. Now, we know about inflammation; we know what it causes and that we like some of what it does; and we know that we can detect certain levels of it. The *Wheel of Fortune* fill in the blanks question is:

W T D ? (What to do?) It does us no good to know there's a Tsunami coming if there is no protection available for us. And the answer is so easy and yet, as I've said before, so hard.

Scrape your knee! Ouch! Put some ointment and a Band-Aid on it and … problem solved. Pull a muscle exercising! Elevate and ice. Tincture of time and you're good as new. Pretty cool prescriptions for acute inflammation. Now here comes the toughie. Smoke, take in high sugars daily, pay no attention to high blood pressure, avoid peaceful time for you, and guess what? Nuttin! That's right: Nuttin, honey. Just like the cereal. You can't feel your arteries being stomped on or inflammation's sending its angry proteins throughout your body until you're looking up at the ceiling in an emergency room—if you're lucky. We can go from vertical to horizontal in a nanosecond. Trust me on this as I have had way too many personal nanoseconds in my search for reducing inflammation.

Now I promised that protecting and ameliorating chronic inflammation would be tough and here it comes. There is no single pill or exercise that will do it for you. The treatment has to begin in your mind and become a daily habit. Yes, you'll screw up and fall off the wagon, so to speak. But just hop back on. I'm a big believer in the old axiom, "Perfect is the enemy of Good." Don't make your life miserable being perfect. Have a ball and enjoy life comfortably with Good. But make no mistake; this path to protection really does require daily commitment, a mantra, an index card, a smart phone reminder, or whatever will help you to stay the course.

I know you've heard these principles a thousand times, but please let me add a few twists. Exercise is absolutely prescription number one. But don't moan or sigh. There's some good news. The facts are that daily exercise is a key factor to wellness and reducing inflammation. Now, exercise is also inflammatory. Yes, it's inflammatory. And again, the key is moderation. I know that I'll get hate letters, but the truth is that marathons are killers and not the least bit good for you. Gotta run one? Fine. Get in shape and run it. Put the medal up in a place where you can see it and say, "Damn, that took a hell of a lot out of me!" Because it sure did. Walk every day? Go for it. But how much exercise, Doc? Fifteen minutes a day … thirty minutes would be ideal. You don't have fifteen minutes? Let me write you a prescription for a new life. Everyday movement in yoga, Pilates, tai chi, etc. are probably the best. This type of exercise reduces heart attacks, increases recovery after heart illness, reduces stress, and so much more and … guess what? We haven't a clue why they work so well. Next in line is resistance training. This can be done with hands, free weights, machines, or just your own body weight. Now I know there's someone out there saying, "I really don't want big muscles." So here's my promise. Work the program and if you end up with huge muscles, please sue me! In forty years, it's never happened to me. I work out seven days a week and when I try to show my wife my "Guns," it takes her ten minutes to stop laughing. Resistance training helps to avoid the muscle loss we experience with aging. Please remember that muscle is a major source for using sugar. And, of course, muscle does all that fabulous stuff like dancing, rowing, and bike riding—not to mention helping to keep us upright so we don't fall and fracture our hips. Exercise/movement is just the single most satisfying gift that you can give to your body. Enough said. Now let's follow the commercial slogan and "Just Do It."

I don't wanna, but I gotta. I have to talk about pills and inflammation. We have become brainwashed to the concept that for every malady, there is a pill. And indeed, we are correct. But that doesn't mean they are necessarily good for us or without risk. And, by "pills," I mean prescription drugs, over the counter meds, and supplements. And every drug/herb/supplement company has us believing that their pill is the best and will cure us. Remember the truism that "Everyone is entitled to their own opinion BUT NOT their own facts." So here's a fact that I hope you never forget. Last year we in the medical professions killed more than 110,000 people with medication errors. Yup, lots more people than we lost in all of the Vietnam War. What's that I hear you saying? "I'm sticking to herbs and supplements!" Yes, your odds are better, but there's no one keeping close tabs on them. And how are they interacting with your prescription meds? The only difference between a pill and a poison is the dose. So when offered a pill, you should always be asking: "Will this improve my life, help me to live longer, not interact negatively with my other meds, have side effects or complications?" In other words: "Can I live as well without it?" But are there pills that can help with inflammation? Certainly. From a prescription standpoint, steroids are king. They specifically target sites of inflammation and quiet them down. Ask anyone with severe arthritis, a raging poison ivy rash, or severe asthma attack. Steroids are amazingly effective but not without a price. They also cause swelling, water retention, elevated sugar, poor sleep, bone loss, and wicked irritability. There are many newer anti-inflammatories but they too affect blood counts and our livers. And when it comes to anti-inflammatories, let's not forget our old faithful standbys such as aspirin and ibuprofen (Aleve, Motrin). Great anti-inflammatories but did I mention gastrointestinal bleeding? Scared? Good! Medicines are great but clearly over used.

Supplements can also be used for inflammation. These are more commonly recommended when your symptoms and labs confirm chronic inflammation. The list of anti-oxidants (which clean up excess free radicals) is never-ending but some of the more useful and widely studied are Omega 3 (fish oil), CoQ10 (excellent), Vitamin C, Vitamin D-3, Glutathione, SAM-e (S-adenosylmethionine), B complex, vitamins, DHEA (dehydroepiandrosterone), Magnesium, and Curcumin. If you take all the supplements available for anti-inflammation, you have no room left for a bite of brownie ala mode! An excellent resource for information on inflammation and supplements can be found at www.LEF.org (Life Extension Foundation). This is an extremely creditable resource.

If you never lifted a weight, ventured to a single yoga class, or took another supplement, you will still do the best for your body by what you put into it. I am a strong believer in the fact that there is no such thing as a "bad food". (That includes a Krispy Kreme donut!) Only too much of it. And, for the most part, that's absolutely true. One exception: tobacco. Ain't a darn thing good about tobacco in any form for your body. No, not even the new "vapor" cigarettes. So, to simplify eating in general, my mantra is: "If it's white, don't bite and if it's green, it will make you lean." Have ice water with every meal and eat off a seven-inch diameter plate. Voila! Even I can remember that. Every two weeks is cheat day. Did you say pizza, baked potato, ice cream? Count me in. And here's a good-news quiz: What has the highest anti-oxidant level of anything and it starts my day? Good old coffee. Amazing but true…. Coffee and fish as a mainstay in your diet and leave the rest to meditation and quiet walks.

In closing my comments in this chapter, let me pass along

some aphorisms that I have picked up along the way. They tie in to what we've been saying. And like The Letterman Show, I'd like to give you my Top Ten. Enjoy:

#10 If your time ain't come, not even your doctor can kill you.

#9 We make ourselves sick by worrying about our health.

#8 To live long, live slowly.

#7 What you don't take can't hurt you.

#6 Just because your doctor has a name for your condition, doesn't mean they know what it is.

#5 If a food is good for you, it won't taste as good as ice cream.

#4 Most conditions will improve without medical intervention.

#3 Many conditions that do not improve without intervention, will not improve *with* intervention.

#2 Effective medicine consists of recognizing those conditions for which interventions are appropriate.

#1 If you think you're not well, you are (not well), and no doctor should tell you otherwise.

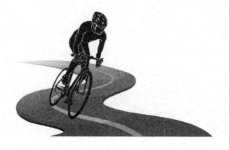

Chapter 4

# *Eating and Drinking: It All (Eventually) Becomes Us*

L et's have some fun. I am going to write this chapter (as
well Chapter 5 which deals with fitness and Chapter 7
titled "Vices") without any direct input from Tom. He and I
have certainly discussed these topics in the past but not recently and not with respect to this book. After I have written
and have done some polishing of what I have to say in this
chapter as well as in Chapters 5 and 7, I will hand it over to
Tom for an analysis of what I have to say. This should prove
interesting because he has no idea that I intend to put him
on the spot. One thing we can all be sure of is that we will
receive a candid and cogent response from the Doc on what
I am doing regarding food and drink intake and other things
and see if it is consistent with aging deliberately.

Now, I want to say something about semantics. You will
notice that I have labelled this chapter "Eating and Drinking."

I did *not* title it "Diet." I think the word *diet* is a far better term, but I chose not to use it in order to draw attention to it. You see, the nutritional definition of diet relates to the *sum* of foods and liquids ingested by an organism. It does not relate to a specific prescribed type of eating and drinking regimen that is specifically designed to have the user shed pounds or control certain substances in response to excessive weight, allergies, conflicts with medications, etc. That said, I think, for many of us, *diet* is associated with the concept of "going on a diet" of some type—usually to shed excess weight. I want us to get away from that concept—at least for this discussion—and think of diet in its macro sense. In other words and turned into the form of a question:

What do you intend to ingest regularly for the rest of your life?

As important a question as this one is, it does beg another: Is your answer to my lead-in question consistent with aging deliberately (i.e., healthily)? And the answer to the follow-up question is, for me, two-fold: Diet is consistent with aging deliberately if it (1) avoids or at least limits essentially unhealthy stuff and (2) it embraces ... here's that word yet again ... *balance.*

**Here is a list of some of the things that I believe are essentially unhealthy (for reasons I may not even remember anymore) and that I generally try to avoid:** [10]

**Soda of virtually any kind.** Yes, I am talking about everything from Mountain Dew to Coke. I don't care if it's diet

---

[10] Remember: This is my list. I am well aware that this is not going to work for everyone. The key, I believe, is to give some real thought and planning into what you take in each day for nourishment and purely for pleasure. Have I mentioned balance lately?

or sugared; I simply don't drink it. I suppose an argument could be made for ginger ale—especially to deal with minor tummy issues—and that is OK, but this is *my* list and consistency here is almost as important as balance. So I stay away from this stuff, period. I have been told a whole bunch of times: Come on, Steve, lighten up! What harm is there going to be in having a Diet Pepsi once in a while. For me, it is sort of a slippery slope thing. Since I believe that all soda is not good for us, I simply can't be comfortable with having one occasionally because its harmful effects will be minimal. I trust myself but there is always that nagging thing in the back of my mind (like there was with smoking) that one could lead to another then another and then another until I am back in the habit again. Paranoid? Probably not. Overly cautious? Well, maybe. But it works for me and I certainly don't miss soda or lots of other stuff on my list.

**Traditional desserts.** You know what I mean. I'm talking doughnuts, pie, cake, pudding, and all the rest of that sugary sweet, doughy, creamy stuff that follows a wonderful dinner or cries out from the fridge to be the main course of a midnight snack. Need I also mention Twinkies, Ho-Hos, donuts, cupcakes, and all those other processed and packaged-in-cellophane treats that have virtually no nutritional value yet have a shelf life of a thousand years (and probably longer). My avoidance of dessert foods has, believe it or not, been a source of some controversy for me. As a naval officer, college department head and dean, friend, and family member, I have attended *lots* of birthday, graduation, wedding, and other types of celebrations and parties. And the overwhelming majority of these include celebratory sweets—especially cakes. When declining an offered slice, I have seen every unhappy emotion—from disappointment to resentment—in the eyes of the partiers surrounding me. And of course, the old refrain kicks in again: "One piece isn't going to kill you, Steve." I used to give in—especially at military celebrations—and eat a small piece. Then, for a while, I would accept a small piece of whatever they were distributing and then sneak off to a safe place to unceremoniously dump it. But not anymore. Eating things I no longer enjoy, sneaking, and dumping are simply not terms and words that are consistent with aging deliberately. Being gracious and not needlessly offending folks is also important. So, I have found that a simple and friendly but resolute "no thank you" usually works just fine. I know, I know.… Some of you may be saying "I don't see the *balance* here, Steve." But I would argue that, taken in a macro sense, there is balance to my diet. I hope to demonstrate how and why in the paragraphs to follow.

**Candy.** Just about any type of candy is full of sugar and/or carbs and is a big problem. Consequently, I avoid it. But what do we do about chocolate which is the basic ingredient for just about every candy bar I can think of? Well, chocolate is just a tad bit complicated because, while a lot of the chocolate out there is *milk* chocolate and about as bad for you as it is incredibly tasty, a lot of it is *dark* chocolate which has many health benefits. Tom has been encouraging me to eat dark chocolate for years now. I still have not made it part of my diet and I am not even sure why—habit, I guess. In any case, I am going to ask you not to follow my lead here and do what Tom suggests: Go ahead and have a nice piece of dark chocolate as healthy and tasty treat.

**Whole-fat dairy products.** Here I am talking about foods ranging from whole milk to ice cream (which also obviously fits into the preceding category as well) to regular cottage cheese to most other types of cheeses. (Note that I said "most" cheeses, not all. See ... a glimmer of balance.)

**Most red meat.** This is a more recent development—almost no mammal meat since about 2009. Lots of nuances here. First, when I say meat I am basically talking about the flesh (mostly water, protein, and fat) of living creatures. So ... if I eat the flesh of a cow or a pig or a chicken or a turkey or a salmon, I am eating *meat*. I, for one, have grown just a little tired of hearing people think that vegetarians don't eat cows but do eat chicken and/or fish. Meat is meat and I simply don't eat *mammal* meat. As a rule .... So are there exceptions? Yes. If a hunter friend kills an elk and asks me if I would like some of the meat, I will enthusiastically say "Yes!" No farm-raised food; I'm talking wild, lean, delicious, protein-rich venison. The next exception is the friends-who-have-prepared-a-lovely-meal-including-stripsteaks-and-have-forgotten-your-dietary-norm situation. In such cases, I follow his holiness the Dalai Lama's lead and go with the flow. Having a small portion of steak is certainly *not* going to kill me; I can handle this possibly one-time-a-year exception. Moreover, as a rule, no traditional burgers, bacon, sausage, hot dogs, ham, lamb, deer, squirrel ... you get the idea. Does that mean I never eat burgers, bacon, or sausage? Nope. I simply substitute: turkey and/or chicken or beans substitute very nicely for many of these items, and I love 'em!

**Alcohol.** No, this is really not on my list of things that I avoid, but it seems like as good a place as any to discuss it. I will also have something to say about alcohol in chapter 7 on Vices. If there are three things related to food and drink intake (aka "diet") that demand balance, they are sugar, salt, and alcohol. For those of us who have no fundamentally acute problems with these three things[11] when used in moderation, we can derive a great deal of pleasure in allowing reasonable amounts of these substances into our bodies. Tom will have much more to say about all three—especially sugar and salt—later, but I want to briefly discuss alcohol here. Here is what I think I know. There is a substance in red wine called resveratrol that is really good for cardiovascular health. So ... most wellness experts will support drinking a glass (for women) or two (for men) most days.[12] I am such a firm believer in resveratrol that I take it in a 250 mg capsule each morning. I don't drink red wine much anymore mainly because I only really enjoyed it when having it with a meal featuring red meat. (Yes, I am traditional in that regard.) Since I eat almost no mammal meat anymore, my red-wine drinking circumstances are rare. My drink of choice is either vodka and lemonade or white wine. These both present problems for me: the lemonade (even organic, no-corn syrup lemonade) is loaded with sugar and vodka is alcohol without the benefit of resveratrol; white wine also is resveratrol free and alcoholic and ... tends to go down far too easily and quickly for me. I remain mindful of these facts and do keep balance in mind ....

**Many kinds of cooking oil and spreads.** I know that trans-fat comes in many processed types of foods, and various kinds of cooking oils are full of it. Bottom line: **All trans-fat is the enemy—no exceptions—avoid it completely whether**

---

[11] Folks who have to deal with diabetes, serious cardiovascular issues, alcoholism, and other significant health issues that completely restrict or significantly limit ingestion of these things have to play by a different set of rules if they wish to remain healthy and age deliberately.

[12] Sorry, ladies, the rules for safe alcohol consumption are different for men and women. Tom knows the science behind this and will discuss it later. It's only fair to know why the rules are different for something that is really a pleasure.

**in cooking oil or in anything else.** I learned fairly recently that safflower oil and canola oil are fairly low in good fats and, while they normally do not contain trans-fat, they are full of other types of fat that should be limited. They are often found in spreads, too. I will have more to say later about the cooking oils and spreads that are actually beneficial.

**Now for the (mostly) really good stuff.** Now that we have discussed the things that I believe all of us need to avoid or significantly limit, what should we focus on for really good and deliberate eating and drinking and, consequently, health-ful, deliberate aging? Well, there are thousands of things we could discuss here, but I am going to stay with what *I* think I know and will leave the rest to Tom who I am challenging here to discuss in several pages of healthy commentary later in this chapter. Once again, at the risk of sounding repetitive, I am going to repeat it … BALANCE. Sure, for most of us, oats are a really good thing to eat[13], but do we want to fill up on oats at every meal? I sure hope not.

**Veggies.** By now, this should be obvious, but not all veg-gies are created equal. I am certain that a nice helping of el dente steamed broccoli trumps any kind of corn any time. Kale is much better for us than iceberg lettuce. Carrots top celery and yams and sweet potatoes rule over conventional potatoes. (Leave those skins on!) . My rule of thumb with veggies is to try to go local, in season, and lightly cooked (steamed) if at all. Some may be surprised to learn that fresh-frozen veggies are often more nutritious than "fresh" ones that may have been sitting around in storage units, trucks, and markets for quite a while before being eaten. (Peas are a good example of this

---

[13] Note, however, there is that pesky gluten issue that I am going to defer to Tom to discuss.

phenomenon.) I know that tomatoes are fruits, but I am going to mention them here because …. I am a tomato junkie. And, guess what… tomatoes are actually even better for you when they are cooked.

**Fruits.** Did I mention that tomatoes are fruits…? Olives are fruits, too. As far as I am concerned, the more of these that I eat, the better. Other really healthy favorites of mine include cantaloupe, bananas (be sure they are not overripe), blueberries, strawberries, blackberries, cranberries,[14] and plums. I am confident that some fruit is really good for us but *lots* isn't. I think the key word with most fruits is—once again—*balance*. I know that some of you may be thinking: "Is he off his rocker?! We need to eat as much fruit as possible. It's a great source of all kinds of things that we need!" Well, there is a lot of truth to that. The problem with many types of fruits, however, is that they are loaded with glucose … yup, sugar. And sugar in quantities above 20 grams per day is a problem. Eating lots of fruit can get you to that threshold number rather quickly. So go ahead and enjoy the wonderful tastes and health benefits of fruit; just keep that 20-grams-of-sugar-per-day standard in mind.[15] We all need to be careful with fruit *juices* as well. Most contain very high levels of sugar and some, like V-8, are quite high in sodium.

**Bulk foods.** If you have an opportunity to buy food in bulk (you know the drill… there is often a big container of,

---

[14] I think there are purists out there who might argue that berries are not really fruits. To me, this is not worth arguing over. Classify them any way you want, but please enjoy them!

[15] Sure, go ahead and break the 20 grams barrier from time to time if you want to; just don't make a habit of it. And do yourself a favor and do a little research on the average amount of sugar that is contained in various quantities of your favorite fruits so that you can keep track.

say, grits or oats or barley at your health-food store), do it. The reason is that, by doing so, you are probably getting only the food you want and no additives. Bulk buying is also a good way to reduce unnecessary packaging.

**Snacks**. Dill pickles, pepperoncini, celery, carrots, radishes, popcorn, nuts (especially almonds, cashews, and walnuts), and seeds.[16]

**What about saturated fats?** I had been in the all-saturated-fat-is-our-enemy mode for at least a couple of decades. Recently, I have been trying to shed this simplistic view and get with the science—as I understand it. My take is that the bottom line now is that some saturated fats—once again, taken in a balanced manner—are really quite good for you as they can help to lower bad cholesterol and raise the good HDLs. **Eggs, avocados, coconut oil, and walnut oil all have their share of saturated fat, but ... it's good stuff in the right quantities ... of course.**

**Fish.** I eat quite a bit of fish—especially salmon, sardines, tuna, grouper, cod, walleye, whitefish, and cat fish as well as shellfish such as mussels, shrimp, and clams. Most folks would say this is a good thing and, generally, they would be right. Unfortunately, nothing—especially diet—is easy. Many fish contain some levels of mercury and mercury is not a healthy substance to take into your body. Other fish such as swordfish and shark are, in my view, caught in unsustainable numbers and, consequently, are in long-term peril of being wiped out. Other species such as cat fish and salmon are often farm-raised which is also problematic. In any case, I believe that eating

---

[16] Full disclosure here: I am a chip lover—the saltier the better. So ... I do indulge myself but with a careful eye on the saturated fat, calorie, and sodium content.

many types of fish in reasonable amounts is a good thing, and I intend to continue to do so.

**Poultry.** I eat my fair share of chicken and turkey … and then some.[17] Once again, this is not without its issues. Commercial poultry farming in the United States is not only problematic because of the way the animals are treated as they are raised and processed but also in the huge amounts of pollutants (i.e., manure) that is produced and often ultimately found in important bodies of water. Chesapeake Bay's significant pollution problems are due, in large part, to the commercial poultry business. I eat and sleep better by purchasing organic chicken and turkey whenever possible. It is pricey but more than worth the extra expense.

**Some breads.** As you know by now, I am aware of the gluten issue. I do not believe, however, that gluten is an issue of concern for me. So I count my lucky stars and eat about one good-sized slice per day—usually as toast with breakfast—and virtually always rye which I have recently started making myself.

**Some dairy.** I love butter but I have tried to avoid it as much as possible for about ten years now. I have mellowed a bit on this and do use small amounts of butter with olive oil mixtures for a spread on my toast a couple of times a week; otherwise, I go with dry toast. And I do occasionally add moderate amounts to the mix when I cook. No big deal. I am also a big fan of low-fat cottage cheese and low-fat yogurt—both tasty, full of good stuff, and even relatively filling.

**Water—LOTS of it.** I'll steal Tom's thunder here. He says we should all drink eight eight-ounce glasses each day. I do not

---

[17] I always remove the skin and as much fat as possible from the meat and try to go organic/free range as much as possible.

do this regularly (see the chapter on vices), but I know that he is right on target on this and I am trying to be better with this.

**Coffee and tea.** I drink between one and three cups of black coffee virtually every day (almost always in the morning). I think one cup is really good for me; two (my norm) is probably OK; and three or more … maybe not so good. Tea (always green with some honey) is a real favorite. I probably don't drink enough of this—only three to five cups a week. I really have no reason not to drink more tea. So, I think I will make a point of doing so.

**Organics.** There has been all kinds of discussion about the possible benefits of organic foods. I, for one, am sold. The idea of eating chicken that is antibiotic free and had a pretty good free-range life just up until the end sits pretty well with me. Eating potatoes that are not filled with pesticides or other harmful substances is also comforting and… healthy. That said, I am not going to be particularly vehement in my encouraging you to go organic whenever possible. The reason for my hesitation to be more of an advocate is, at this time at least, simple: expense. Let me give you an example—it may be an extreme one, but it does speak directly to my point. As I write this section, it is the Wednesday before Thanksgiving and I have been back home for only about two hours since picking up the organic turkey and some other organics that I bought at a Whole Food store some fifty minutes away. (Not real pleased about the questionable environmentally unsound act of driving that far for groceries, but I do not make a practice of it.) The cost of the turkey… just about four bucks a pound! Is this a luxury that everyone can afford, let alone a weekly practice for purchasing all foods? Certainly not. So … my recommendation is to do what you can afford and find a balance that suits you, your health and nutrition goals, and your budget.

**Home-Juiced Veggies.** I can't think of many things that are better to eat/drink than fresh organic vegetables that you juice right at home. I especially like to start with a carrot juice base and go from there. There are as many possibilities and combinations here as you can imagine. I highly recommend creating your own home-juiced veggies as often as you can. That said, I also offer this caveat: Be prepared for some expense and lots of clean-up time. We have already discussed the relatively high price for organic foods (reduced dramatically if you grow your own, of course). Juicing is time consuming, however, and cleaning up is a bit of a pain[18]—especially if you don't have lots of spare time.

I have a couple of oh-by-the-ways to close this chapter. They are things you have heard before, but they are worth mentioning here (again). First, since it is almost a requirement to allow some oils into your diet for salads, cooking, and other things, why not do yourself a big favor and use coconut oil? There are other types out there that will do you far more good than harm, but this one is my favorite. It's even good to rub on your skin! Second, and maybe most important, try—and I mean *really* try—not to stuff yourself with food at meal time or at any time. I mean this. Pushing yourself away from the table while you still feel like you could probably eat more can mean the difference between maintaining a healthy weight and becoming obese. The fact is that, if you stop shoveling it in for just a little while, your brain will catch up with your tummy and you will feel like you have had plenty to eat. Just keep in mind the proportions of food Tom advocates and stay close to those amounts and you should do really well. A third

---

[18] Your juicing equipment needs to be thoroughly cleaned each time you use it. The good news is that the residue from your juicing is great for composting.

thing to keep in mind is to consider eating several mini meals during the day versus the traditional big three. This practice—at least two or three times a week—can really help in weight management. Finally, consider fasting—say, from dawn to dusk—maybe a couple of times a month; and, when you do finally eat, take it easy—especially on the carbs.

So enough for *my* discussion of diet. It is obviously very important, but it is not all there is to looking and feeling great. And please keep in mind, once again, that what Tom and I recommend in this chapter is not written in stone. Pick, choose, and add what you think will work best for you. Just be honest with yourself and, if you do cheat once in a while, don't stress over it. Just remember to get back on track and stay there for a while. Eating and drinking wisely will not guarantee a small waist line and good health, but doing so will serve as an excellent *part* of a healthy lifestyle that will keep you feeling well and… aging deliberately. Now it is time for Tom to respond to what I just fessed up to and to add some additional comments.

Take it away, my Friend.

I never thanked my banker when he handed me my mortgage payment book, so I'm not sure why I should thank Steve for asking me to contribute to this chapter. But I will thank him because he has allowed me to add comments about a subject that he is not only passionate about but also extremely knowledgeable about as well. Now, some of you might expect that, as a physician, I would begin with a lot of pomp about credentials and various studies touting this point or that. But the fact is that we, as health professionals in general, know practically nothing about nutrition and exercise. Tough to believe? Well these areas are not part of the medical school curriculum, for starters. Want more proof? Take a look at most physicians with their excruciatingly long hours, stress-filled days, and horribly unhealthy lifestyles. Looking well nourished, fit, and frisky…? Nope. Not one of my personal physicians is close to the health picture of Steve.

But before Steve gets too big of a head, please let me point out some critical points. First, Steve is in the top 1% of Americans—health wise—for his age. He not only looks great but his performance levels are those of a truly fit athlete. Steve's lifestyle and nutrition guidelines are untouchable. There is not a single word of advice that he has given that I could dispute.

Whoa! If that's all there is, then I should end the chapter right here. But I must let you in on a little secret. I'm seventy-one years old and have survived a ton of medical catastrophes. I also gave my body a gauntlet of abuses and, to an extent, still do. So what's my point? Simply this: Steve treats his body as a temple. And it shows. I tend to treat my body like a drive-in diner! Now please don't get me wrong. I'm not advocating my lifestyle (although it has gotten me past seventy), nor am I setting Steve's as your goal. (Mainly because most of us can't make it to his level. I want to slam dunk a basketball in Madison Square Garden, but that ain't happening in my lifetime.)

The point is this. I hope that all of us can try to improve our lifestyles every day. Yes, *every* day. To illustrate, I take out a 3x5 card each night and write out one goal for the next day. The goals are always simple and usually doable…not vague crap like "lose weight." What the heck does that mean, anyway? Or, what about "exercise?" Really?! Means nothing without meat, substance? So my goals might include something like "no diet sodas today." Or maybe "twenty minutes of interval rowing" in the morning. How about "compliment my wife" or "ask the cashier at the grocery store what he likes about his job—not just "How are you?" With my 3x5 card in my pocket (yes, you do have to write it down), I'm off for the day's adventures. I think you get that the trick is not only to make a point of doing something special to improve one's life even in a relatively simple way each day, but also taking the time to think about the fact that each moment of each day *is* something special and then taking action on that fact.

What's this have to do with nutrition, exercise, and all the rest? Well, in my opinion, all components of aging can be fun and fulfilling. But you must have a map to get started and stay on course. And that may require a huge change in your *mind* style to positively affect your lifestyle. And, to quote Yogi Berra (why not, everyone else does and I doubt he really said much of anything that has been printed): "If you don't change your direction, you're gonna end up where you're heading." Atta boy, Yogi!

So let's get to the "meat and potatoes," as they say. Once again, I must absolutely concur with every word of Steve's advice. Absolutely perfect. But what I'd like to do is hit you with some thoughts and facts about both nutrition and exercise for those of us not quite at Steve's level. (I will have even more to say about physical fitness at the end of Chapter Five.) For the "wannabees," "mightbees," "couldbees," and even "ain't-never-gonnabees," this is for you.

First, as you know, this is your life and you have the gift of choosing how to play it. The bottom line that we never, nor should we ever, forget is that we are all here to live and die. Notice that I did not say "pass away"; I said *die*. Will a donut make a difference in that fact? Not on your life (every bit of pun intended). Will a donut a day make a difference? You betcha! The heavy carb load will beat your arteries, promote hypertension and stroke, and help you to cruise right into Cancer Bayou and Heart Attack Lagoon. So, we'll tend to stick with the donut analogy, even though the concept applies to alcohol, smoking, drugs, etc. In any case, in attempting to create and maintain a healthy, sane life style, the issue is basically this: How much is too much? Well, for some things, the answer is easy. Tobacco, NONE. Not a damn thing good to say about anything going into your mouth and/or lungs than good, clean air. But when it comes to life choices, here's a secret that we physicians don't want you to know. We don't have a clue as to what works best for each of you. So help me, that's true. Yes, we throw around lots of big words and quote the science but none of it fits each of you like a well-made shirt. You bet. Terms? Sure, here are just a few: BMR—basal metabolic rate; EAT—exercise activity thermogenesis (What?! It's just a fancy phrase for measurement of calories burned from exercise); TEF—thermal effect of food (this is the calories burned from eating... Yes, from simply ingesting food). But none of these and a bunch more of such measurements will tell me how much broccoli you should eat. They won't help me to figure out what exercise program you should be on or how often you should work out. Man, what a mess! Now I can fake it as well as any doc, but the fact of the matter is that the real skipper of your boat, your lifestyle, your weight, your intake, your exercise—your overall health care—is YOU. I know that you didn't need to hear that 'cause you have known that for years. It's just hard to put all of it together in a neat package that you can change and fit to what suits you and your health best.

So here are a few principles to guide you. Starting with this: The mind is *numero uno*; be ready to use it to help you commit to the Yogi principle and to be set to make small deliberate changes. No, not to live longer, although that certainly may be an outcome. But to live BETTER. "What does that mean?" I hope you're asking. Well, "better" for me means less pain, more energy, and avoiding stroke, cancer, and heart problems. (No guarantees, mind you, but the key is giving yourself the best shot possible while keeping a sane lifestyle that you can live with.) Sound good? Please remember that this applies to YOUR head, YOUR mind. Sit and put your Yogi plan together. Maybe start with your 3x5 card tomorrow saying nothing more than "fill in a card each day." And your goal…? Perhaps it's more like "heathier to be happier." Maybe it's "healthier to limit my anxiety." Make the change! This really can be, and is, the best life ever. No spin.

Well, I promised diner-style simplicity so here goes. Heads together. Small, deliberate, changes. What are some truthful maxims we can come up with to make this all a little more manageable? In providing a few, let me provide a little more background first. I work in a free clinic in my home town and some of my patients live in boxes or under the bridges. They are "hard ground" folks because that's where most of them sleep. Junk food, alcohol, and drugs are their staples. Those products make them feel good. I mean really good. Broccoli doesn't. They live simple lives but they have the same desires as you and I have: an ounce of pleasure in the day and avoidance of pain. I offer them (and, of course, you) these maxims:[19]

> Eat every meal from a 7-inch plate, but first
> drink water—don't wait!

---

[19] You will probably detect some repetition here with regard to my comments in Chapter 3 but that's OK by me.

It it's white, just don't bite.

But don't say "No." Just say "Whoa!"

Do fifteen minutes of exercise, and a healthy
life you'll realize.

If you don't buy it, you won't have to try it.

You are what you think, so give a hand and
a wink.

I've gotta tell you the answer to the question that's burning
in your mind right now: No, I have never had formal poetry
or rhyming classes. Amazing, isn't it?! Well, maybe not so
amazing. But here's the gist. These are easy guidelines and
they work like this. First, always *eat from a 7-inch plate*. Fill
it with a cheeseburger if you want, but 7 inches is it. Drink
eight to twelve ounces of ice water BEFORE each meal. This
will release a hormone (leptin) that makes you feel full and
you'll actually burn calories to raise the temp of the ice water
to body temp (98.6F).

*White foods* are usually chock full of carbohydrates. Now
I'm a carboholic. I'll step on your back for ice cream or a
baked potato. Better yet, give me both! Unfortunately, most
carbs today are weak in energy; they also raise insulin too high
and then cause it to come crashing down creating the need
for more. As a guide, for people like me who vacuum in the
carbs, forty grams of carbs per meal is reasonable, particularly
if you're diabetic (like me). The key is to add as much fiber as
you can with each meal. Thirty to fifty grams of fiber per day

is the minimum. I always have to add commercial fiber such as Fiber One, Metamucil, or MiraLAX to help things along … if you know what I mean.

I still stick with the axiom that there are no "bad foods"— just too much of some. But if you think you can always just say "NO" to some "baddy," I'll yell "Liar, liar, pants on fire!" For me, I guarantee you that I'll have a donut within a month. Now it may only be half a donut and only once a month, but damn, they taste too good for me to never eat again. And that donut sure won't keep me from the Olympics. My clumsy un-coordinated body will, but I can't blame a donut. Again, the point is not to fight yourself. You're going to trip and you're going to splurge, but you can start all over again with the next meal that enters your body. Enjoy life by *not saying "No, No, No." Just say "Whoa."* Whoa stands for "maybe tomorrow," or "Do I really need that?" or "OK, but maybe just half a serving." I can live with any of those, but I can't deal with "No, never again for me. I'd rather die than eat another square of dark chocolate." Oh, that's right; I'm gonna die some day! My goal is to die with a smile and as healthy as I can be.

*Fifteen minutes of exercise?* Yup, that's all you need to do. But do it every day. There is nothing better that you can do for yourself. Seriously, nothing. Now if you want the perfect exercise routine, it's simple. Exercise before each meal. You see, exercising lowers insulin and insulin inflames your arteries. And that's worse than hitting a cop car. Exercise lowers insulin and sugar in your blood so it makes sense to do it before each meal. But Hey! Let's get real here. In most cases, that just ain't gonna happen. At least not in my life. So what's a real schedule? Everyday exercise for healthy living. It's like paying your health insurance premium. It keeps illness at bay. An exercise routine should include stretching (I do mine in bed when I wake and it takes about five minutes. I hold a pose or stretch for five breaths); resistance training (lifting your body weight by doing pushups, squats, pullups, and so many others or by using hand/arm weights and/or leg weights); and aerobics (walking, jump rope, jumping jacks, biking, hula hoop, etc.). Notice that I left out running. Sorry. Now, if you're a runner of years, go for it. But as we age, joints just don't do well being beat on. And here's a kicker. Yoga and rowing are two of the best exercises around. But like all endeavors, make sure you get expert instruction first to avoid injury.

*If you don't buy it, you won't have to try it.* I know what you're thinking again. He's a genius! No, not really, but the king of the obvious. I'm really just hammering home a point that a major part of what goes in our bodies is via our grocery cart. So there really is validity to comparing looking into our carts to looking into our arteries. (Gross, I know, but true.) When wheeling through the grocery store, stay on the outside where most of the good stuff lies. Hit those veggies hard and even some new stuff whose names you can't pronounce. Add anything to salsa and it's a party! For example, I hate spinach. But I've learned that fried spinach with a tad bit of olive oil, lemon, and even ranch dressing can be yummy. Uh oh, what's that around the corner? Ruffles potato chips! If I don't buy it, I won't try it. But I love them! Where's that "Whoa" rule now when I need it? OK, so buy the individual bag or the small one on the shelf as you check out. (Companies put them there because, in their heart of hearts, they worry that you may need a snack for the ride home!) The enemy is everywhere but we can have some fun beating them at their own game. How about this: "Don't buy *all* of it, so you won't *try* all of it." Because in the history of man, no one has thrown out three-fourths of a bag of Ruffles.

*You are what you think, so give a hand and a wink.* Of all the maxims I've ever heard, this one has the most meaning for me. First, you definitely ARE what you think. Aside from clinical psychiatric disease, how we choose to feel is how we'll be. Just that simple. All of us need to choose to be happy every morning. Bills due, cars broken, overslept, spouse upset, the kids are lazy, and you feel crazy. Doesn't matter. You still get to choose. If the day sucks, it is probably because we *let* it suck. Very basic and very true. Now how do you choose happy? You have to leave YOU. Finding someone else to help is the key. Years ago, in Navy flight school, our drill instructor (a tiger in a U. S. Marine Corps uniform) looked at all of us as cadets and said: "Look left and right. One of you wants to quit today. Be his wingman today and help because tomorrow it may be you in that seat." Same principle isn't it? Help someone.

Steve has reminded me that this book is not going to rival *War and Peace* in length and just about everything else, for that matter. So, here's my wrap up for this chapter. Learn to be comfortable with your dying while you're living every second today. Exercise is not work. It really is a gift that you give to yourself. Food is also such a gift. Choose healthily for everything that passes your lips. It's the long run nutrition that really counts for your wellbeing, not the occasional stumbles that can be so much fun. Enjoy the day by giving it away in what you do to and for others and enjoy your life's journey— for you—and others will follow. Peace, Tom.

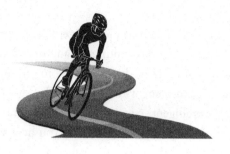

Chapter 5

# *Fitness: Just Move!*

When I am in my nineties, I am going to be more
than merely alive. I am going to be a *Life!*

Most of us would agree that fitness comes in several
forms: physical, mental, emotional, and even financial.
In this chapter, however, I am going to focus on *physical* fitness.
The other forms of fitness are extremely important, of course,
and I will certainly discuss these at other points later in the
book. For now, though, let's talk about physical fitness, and I
will start with a possibly loaded question: How's *yours*?

This is certainly not a question of how far or fast you can
run or how much weight you can lift. After all, for any number of reasons, some of us can't run at all and weight lifting
may not be a good idea for others. Whatever you *can* do to
get yourself into shape and stay there needs to be sanctioned
by your doctor—especially if you have not been active for a
while. So ... for some of you, the substance of this chapter will

actually begin with a commitment to get those muscles in better shape, to work on your endurance, and/or to lose weight.[20] Once you are committed, then you need to see your doc and share your commitment with him/her. The two of you can work out an intelligent, reasonable, fitness program that will not only meet the goals that the two of you have worked out but also will be one that you can sustain. It is very likely that what you come up with will be more than an exercise program; it will be a new way of life. The idea is to get you healthy and keep you there—for good—not to get you hurt.

And I need to double down on this next point: *It is never too late to get started.* Just the other day I was speaking about fitness with a woman who is about fifteen years younger than I am. She was bemoaning the fact that she was in such great shape just a few years ago and now ... she wasn't. She was quick to place the blame for her physical fitness decline on diet and lack of exercise. I just smiled and said, "You can do something about that; you know." She gave me a big smile right back and said, "I *do* know!" And I really do think she is going to get back to fitness and ... feeling better and younger—after she discusses her new fitness plan with her doctor, I hope. More on this later but, for now, just remember that movement—any movement—is a really good thing. Frankly, nothing beats it. *How* you move and how *often* will be something you and your doctor and possibly your personal trainer will develop over time.

---

[20] Checking your weight is not a simple matter of stepping on a scale and feeling good about yourself because you are within some arbitrarily established parameters. For example, I know a number of "skinny fat" people. They don't weigh very much relative to their height, but they lack muscle mass. Their low weight is deceptive; it is masking their generally poor physical condition and ... health.

Now it is time for some more disclosure. When I was in my mid-twenties, I was in graduate school. I also smoked cigarettes and an occasional joint, ate like there was no tomorrow, and did not have a regular exercise program, although I was an excellent softball player and played on several teams. In the course of about two and a half years, I went from weighing about 175 pounds to close to 230 pounds! At the age of twenty-eight, I made myself a promise that I would quit smoking and lose at least fifty pounds before I was thirty and that I would not slip back into my old unhealthy habits. I kicked the smoking and lost about sixty-five pounds before I was twenty-nine. I am not going to tell you that I managed this feat in a particularly healthy way. In fact, I was severely restricting my diet and had gone from cigarettes to chewing tobacco and I still had a great deal to learn about physical fitness training. For me, however, that year was a transition period that led to a commitment to take care of myself and to never stop learning about diet and physical fitness. The result was a total lifestyle change that continues to grow and evolve to this very day. My commitment to physical fitness has evolved—largely as a result of two things: information and some of my physical limitations that I discussed in Chapter 2. Running or playing competitive tennis, for example, are no longer viable options for me. Walking, rowing, resistance training, abdominal and core work, and many other exercise and workout options are. Over time and with the help of the likes of Tom Schneider and Tony Horton, I have developed a program that is not only a great fit for me but also something that I can use and tweak for many years to come. What I do, however, may not be what is right for you. Your doc, your fitness objectives, and your own body will guide you. Just to give you some idea of where I am now, I will provide you with an example of a typical week's fitness activities: [21]

Monday—Morning walk (one-half to one hour or more); ball crunches and bicycles; weight work (curls, military presses, and flies—three to four sets each using twenty-five pound weights); twenty-plus minutes on the elliptical.

Tuesday—Morning bicycle ride (weather permitting) for at least one hour; parts of Tony Horton's P90X abdominal work-out and a couple of planks (one regular and one reverse); three sets of chin-ups (ten to twelve per set); twenty-plus minutes on the rowing machine.

Wednesday—Morning walk (one-half to one hour or more); regular sit-ups (usually one set of about seventy-five) and regular crunches (about one-hundred); pushups [22] (four sets of twenty-five); afternoon bike ride (weather permitting) for one hour plus. Stretching in the AM and PM.

Thursday—Morning bike ride (weather permitting) for one hour plus; rowing with machine for half an hour or more;

---

[21] No week—or day, for that matter—is ever the same, but I do try to do something in three main categories almost every day: resistance training, cardio/calorie burning, abdominal/core work. I also have the luxury of being able to work out at just about any time of the day since I am no longer working regular hours and have assembled a very nice home gym. And, please remember, this is only my example; your own regime will develop over time.

[22] I love pushups because, if done correctly, they are really good for you and so easy to do—just about anywhere. There are also many types of them. My go-to push up involves the use of risers for my hands and placing my toes on an exercise ball. These are great for both resistance training and core work.

planks, ball crunches, and oblique crunches; weight work similar to Monday; twenty-plus minutes on the elliptical.

Friday—Morning walk (one-half to one hour) on a tread mill varying speeds and degrees of inclination;[23] regular sit ups; dips (four sets of thirty-five); twenty-plus minutes on the elliptical.

Saturday—Morning canoeing or kayaking (weather permitting) for one to two hours; parts of Tony Horton's P90X ab workout; chin ups; elliptical for twenty minutes.

Sunday—Walk in the morning for an hour; about fifty push-ups; about fifty ball crunches. Stretching in the AM and PM. Or … sometimes—especially when I have had a relatively strenuous workout schedule during the previous week—I simply take the day off.

As I said before, this sort of a routine is not for everyone, but it does work for me. Some weeks are a little more rigorous and others not so much. There are also some things (e.g., shadow boxing, hiking, swimming, recumbent bike, treadmill, etc.) that I also work in, but were just not part of the week's activities that I used as an example. I am also well aware of the fact that some things that I do are simply not an option for some of you. Walking for an hour is obviously not going to work for someone who needs a chair. What I really want to emphasize here is *movement*—whatever type of movement that challenges you and is healthy for you. Let me follow up on this just a bit. I know a few folks who have significant ankle, knee,

---

[23] This is a form of interval work which is really helpful in cardio and calorie burning workouts of any kind. I highly recommend it.

hip, or other issues that severely limit their ability to walk, run, or do many things on their feet. They have discovered, however, that exercising—at times, vigorously—does not have to be something that they only have fond memories of. They have discovered water aerobics and other great exercises that can be done in the pool [24]—thus significantly reducing the wear and tear and pain that they would undergo if attempting to do similar sorts of activities without the support (and the healthy resistance) that the water can provide.

By the way, you may have noticed that there is no yoga in my discussion of physical fitness. There is a reason for this. While I am a strong proponent of yoga for most folks, I am not a practitioner. It is not for want of trying. The fact of the matter is that many yoga poses so negatively impact my arthritis that the pain overwhelms me to the point where I cannot focus on breathing and I end up after the session in far more pain than I began it. I have discussed this with several yoga instructors and each told me that this is not uncommon and that I can focus on the stretching and balancing components of yoga without practicing most of the poses that are part of a typical session or class. So … stretching and balancing exercises it is!

Just a couple more points about physical fitness as a lifestyle. I think my favorite example for those of us who are able

---

[24] Whether we refer to it as water aerobics, aqua fitness, aquatic fitness, or other terms, working out in shallow water, usually in a pool in waist-deep or even deeper water, vertical (non-swimming) exercise can include jogging, yoga, dancing, and all sorts of other aerobic or even non-aerobic exercise. It can be done individually or in groups and is limited only by our imagination and common sense, of course. A simple visit to your local YM/WCA or health club to obtain more information on where and when introductory, intermediate, or even advanced programs may be available can be enough to get you started. And, of course, you can always just go for a swim!

to move around without assistance is the stairway. Whenever possible—even when carrying luggage or backpacks at the airport—I choose the stairs over the escalator or the elevator. I mow the grass at my house. [25] I use a power mower but I do the pushing. I rake the leaves in the autumn; I do not use a blower. Whenever possible, I hang my clothes on the line to dry instead of using the dryer. The fundamental health benefits of simple, routine house and yard maintenance are amazing.

And now a concluding comment about the overall benefits of staying fit—something that I have alluded to previously. For me, physical fitness is the most important component of preventive health care. I realized a long time ago that the healthcare system—such as it is in the United States—is set up to fix us when we are broken in one way or another. Even now there is far more attention paid to taking pills for various health problems as opposed to determining the lifestyle issue that creates the need for the pills. There simply is far more time spent on surgical procedures to fix health problems than time devoted to promoting and supporting lifestyles that prevent the need for surgeries in the first place. Every time a wing or new floor is added to a local hospital or a new emergency clinic is established I find myself thinking: What if our attention were focused on preventing health issues from occurring to begin with instead of all of this *reactive* medicine? We will leave this as a rhetorical question—especially since I am sure you understood and maybe even embraced my point a page or more ago. Keep moving, my friends! 'Nuff said.

---

[25] Full disclosure here. At the time I first wrote this, I was, in fact, mowing my own lawn. But I have since moved to a house on a much larger lot and am preparing for a right knee replacement. So, for now, I am leaving the lawn cutting work to others.

Tom's Take:

Wait a holy second, Steve! Do you really expect me to follow that last section of yours? Really?! After reading your healthy exercise section, I feel like hopping into my hammock for a good one-hour nap. You are amazing! That is one hell of a work load, my young man (and you always will be!). I guess I get to be the slug again in this book. OK, so be it. Don't I wish that I could follow Steve's workout plan … because it truly is ideal. But, for so many of us, time is our main limiting factor. And, with that in mind, here goes for those of us who struggle for even fifteen minutes of breathing time each day.

I must, again, confirm how fantastic Steve's fitness routine is and particularly with his arthritis. And, not to one up him on this point, I do have my share of medical issues and physical limitations of my own—as I pointed out in Chapter 2. So why the hell am I even alive to be writing this today? So help me, I haven't a clue. But I will share some thoughts regarding things that seem to have worked for me. Have a look and enjoy the ones that make sense to you.

Once there was a farmer who had fallen. He went to the monastery and asked the most learned monk what herbs (pills) he should take. The monk looked at the farmer in a kindly way and told him to simply be gentle to himself and everyone with whom he has contact. Hmmmm. Not bad advice. And I guess that's the best summary of what I do for exercise. But first, I want to emphasize that I totally accept Steve's advice that exercise (along with paying close attention to the quantity and quality of the food we eat) is the best medicine. The Schneider rule is this: If I eat, I exercise. That simple … pretty much seven days a week. I'm not interested in either biceps or "love handles" showing. I keep remembering that exercise moves muscles and they, in turn, suck in sugar and thus lower insulin. Remember that both of those (sugar and insulin) are inflaming to our arteries. The good news is that, as it turns out, just fifteen minutes a day can help keep those critters down and in check. Fifteen minutes! Gotta say it again: fifteen minutes! If anyone doesn't have fifteen minutes a day for movement exercise, I need to write you a prescription for "A New Life."

Do I complete fifteen minutes of exercise *every* day? Just about. But occasionally, sometimes, rarely, once in a blue moon—I don't. It's the truth. Too tired, way too achy, no energy, or whatever other excuse I can come up with that morning. They are rare days, but they do happen. How do I excuse myself for such days? I don't. I enjoy the day and make a new, more exciting index card for an exercise plan for the next day. Now for some specifics.

I take some time to get moving in the morning. So, before I get out of bed, I stretch. Now, I could draw or photograph myself doing this, but this is supposed to be a family book so I'll refrain from doing so. Do whatever you like to stretch and hold each position for five breaths. Twist your hips. Pull your knees up to your chest. Reach your hands toward the ceiling. And remember to breathe deeply throughout. Ahhh, stretching complete, I am a tad more awake. Then slowly out of bed and standing at the side of my bed, I take five more good deep breaths. I feel my feet in contact with the floor. Balance is critical to me. By the way, here's a trick that I do and that I highly recommend that you strongly consider doing yourselves. It has the extra bonus of making your family think that you're nuts. It is really great for balance and has saved me a couple of times. During the day, as I am walking, I practice quickly bending my knees like a genuflection. By doing this, I'm training my mind and muscles so that if I do trip and lose my balance, I will automatically collapse my legs. Why does this matter? Because for most of us over sixty falling on our hips from the standing position puts us at high risk of a hip fracture. Mortality is high for those injuries. Studies have shown the efficacy of such "genuflection" practice for those of us in our "mature" years. (And so here I need to acknowledge and give a special thanks to my fourth grade nun, Sister Angela!)

OK, so we know we want to do something every day but what exactly does that entail? So many factors to look at, but first let's recheck something especially important: time. Fifteen minutes of anything that increases our heart rate counts. No, checking out the latest Chippendale or Victoria's Secret calendar doesn't count. Well, I take that back. It *does* count by letting you know that you are still alive. That counts. But your fifteen minutes need to really move muscle. If you can walk aggressively or simply at a moderate pace, that counts. I also ask my patients to concentrate on resistance exercises (using weights, bands, or their own body weight). One simple daily exercise is to do (or work up to doing) one-hundreds: mini squats or jumping jacks or arm rolls (like trying to fly) or pushups (start by pushing up against a wall while standing) or any combination of these. Pick the ones(s) you like and get started. What? You say that your physical condition will let you push yourself (a lot?) more? OK, move it up to thirty or forty-five minutes of exercise. Steve mentioned Tony Horton's workout program and he has at least two great ones. One is fifteen minutes or up to thirty minutes on a great day. P90X is a much more formal program but you can do it at your own speed and up to the amount that works best for you. I really like it. The point is: DO SOMETHING ACTIVE EVERY DAY. Bad ankle today? Do only upper body. Have a headache? Just walk. You are way too smart for me to do any dumbing down on exercise for you. Tons of books, *YouTube*, and so many more resources and guides are available to you. But … what's missing?

I think that most of us at least occasionally exercise by fighting our minds and that may keep us from being fat heads, but it sure isn't helping the rest of our bodies. Our heads can lead us into so many pits of despair. (Watch *The Princess Bride*, one of my favorite movies, sometime to get a good sense of the pits of despair.) Our minds tell us that we will never look like Pierce Brosnan or Julia Roberts. Our muffin top will never go away. Why do we need to tone these muscles, anyway? Blah, blah, blah ….

You get the point. There's always a reason or an excuse to give in to the ever-present enemy: inertia. But now you know the facts. You need muscle to fight the effects of sugar and insulin. What's that you say? You broke your arm? OK then. Just try doing a simple everyday task like getting out of bed with a pathetically wimpy opposite arm and weak core muscles. Or try using crutches following an ankle sprain. Not going to work if you can't support yourself. For so many reasons—many of them involving preparations for unexpected challenges in our lives—we absolutely need to keep our core and strength muscles fit.

Stuff. Gotta take a few lines for stuff. You know, equipment for exercise. Now, you can skip to the next chapter if you still have your high-school Penny's sneakers or Converse high tops. If you are still holding on to these things and even using them, you are pretty set in your ways and unlikely to move on and up. But, if you're like me, you eat up new exercise programs or gear like Oreos. If that's the case, here's what I've learned after having tried 'em all. For safety, all around body fitness, and max calorie burn, you can't beat the Concept 2 rowing machine. And it's pretty much indestructible. I also like a speed jump rope for simplicity. There's also a system that attaches to any door. It's called the TRX system and it's used by the military special forces for conditioning because of its versatility. It's essentially web bands and you use them with your body weight to perform hundreds of fun exercises. The "Total Gym" is also very effective and safe. Notice a theme here? Safe. I'm embarrassed by the number of days I have been down and out because of doing crazy exercises that my twenty-one-year-old mind has convinced my seventy-year-old body to try. For example, I admit to dropping a twenty-five pound dumbbell (Oops, that was me!) weight on my foot. Yup ... a broken toe, not to mention the pain. It happens, but I like to keep such things to an absolute minimum—for me and for you. I like stretch bands for the same reason. They are safe. One last piece of advice: Invest in quality cross trainer shoes. Not running shoes, sandals, socks, barefoot, or ballet slippers. Why not running shoes? Too narrow and ankle twists are too common. Remember: Safe. Did you say that this is all new to you? Never been in a gym? Invest in a certified trainer. Worth every penny.

So please let this be a healthy-future plea. May we all exercise every day. Fifteen, thirty, forty-five minutes of muscle movement because we owe it to ourselves and we're worth it. I may not look as strong or as fit as Steve, but I *do* look as strong and fit as I can be...for me. Here's the key. I consistently find myself answering YES to this essential question: Are you better today than you were yesterday?

Now here's the Big Christmas Present for sticking to all that's been said here. It comes with a Dementia Prevention Package. Read all of the journals on dementia prevention. Know what you'll see? Avoid inflamers such as alcohol, tobacco, and processed sugar. And EXERCISE! There is simply no substitute—no supplements or magic pills from your doc—that can do all that exercise can for overall fitness. And, once again … exercise has been found to be the most consistent factor for dementia prevention.

Excuse me … "What's that, honey?"

Sorry … that's my wife telling me to go work out because I'm way behind on my dementia prevention program. Isn't she cute?!

**An Afterword on Dental Fitness**

In opening this chapter, I noted that the focus would be on *physical* fitness here. In rereading what Tom and I wrote, it struck me that we did not address a key component of physical fitness that is often ignored or not given adequate attention: dental health. Tom did make some excellent points about the importance of flossing in his chapter on Inflammation, but I want to emphasize all of the components of good dental care here. And, in keeping with this chapter's sub-title ("Just Move"), moving hands, wrists, and arms as you brush and floss is definitely required for this—each and every day. While regular visits to your dentist are a must, your dentist and dental hygienist can't manage your dental health alone. You know this, but are you as proactive in your own dental care as you need to be? I slip occasionally by missing a flossing and that is no big deal; it's the regularity of care, however, that is crucial. Paying attention to your mouth, your tongue, your gums, and your teeth will lead to excellent dental health—even in our most advanced years. And, as any dentist or doc will tell you, excellent dental health is a window into your entire body's wellbeing. Happy brushing and flossing, everyone!

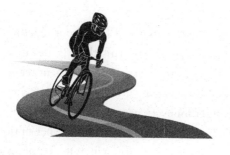

Chapter 6

# The Nuts and Bolts of Vitamins, Herbs, and Supplements

Following a chapter on fitness that focusses on the need for *exercise* to help prevent health issues with a chapter on supplements and other stuff to swallow may seem a bit contradictory. I am not uncomfortable with doing this, however, because there is certainly a place for both in a healthy lifestyle that promotes deliberate aging. I am going to defer to Tom to do the heavy lifting in this chapter, but, by way of introduction, I will say that I do take my share of supplements and even meds. I do so with Tom's support and, in some cases, his strong recommendations.[26] The chart in Appendix II is a

---

[26] I take meds for blood pressure control, GERD, thyroid health, and cholesterol control. I take supplements mostly for cardio health (CoQ10, resveratrol, children's aspirin) and joint support/arthritis control (glucosamine, MSM) plus Vitamin B complex, magnesium, D-3, saw palmetto (for prostate

compilation of what Tom and I have put together as the best supplement regimen *for me*. This chart is meant to be just one example. *Please* do not start any supplement regimen without first thoroughly discussing it with your doctor. Not every supplement is right for every person and almost every supplement has a side effect. Also, there are many other options that are not included in this chart. You will note that many of the supplements that are listed are focused on heart health. This is due to my family history. Finally, keep in mind that, like anything else, supplements and vitamins can differ in quality—another issue to be discussed with your doctor. Now it is Tom's turn.

"PILLS KILLS." Notice the capital letters? And those two words start this chapter! What a downer. But, in my defense my friends, I really have no choice but to drive this point home decisively. Now don't panic. We'll hit all the great vitamins and herbs and bio-identical hormones, but the take-away is that, seriously, pills kills. I'll go so far as to say that, of all the advice that Steve and I have to give, this is the most singularly important. I feel so strongly about this that I am going to share with you two episodes in my life involving pills. The first happened when I was doing triathlons. I was approaching fifty years and had five triathlons under my belt, but the old knees were really aching as I trained for number six. I was well aware of new and exciting and proven beneficial, anti-inflammatory drugs on the

---

health), Krill oil and Omega 3 fish oil, and vitamin K. Yes, I know that it sounds like a lot and my med/sup regimen is not inexpensive, but I am very happy with it. I make the expense along with my exercise equipment credit card payment (formerly fitness center membership) part of each month's budget. Of course, you will want to consult with your doc and your budget before you take the plunge, but I do strongly recommend some supplement program to augment a healthy diet and even to help you sleep better.

market. I decided to give one—Celebrex—a try. This was a great drug and personally proven prior efficacy on my creaky skeleton. In from a long run, dehydrated, and aching, I popped a Celebrex. Two sips of water and I was out ready to play with the kids. That evening, dinner wasn't settling well and nausea progressed to fever and big time tummy pain. Hours later after scans and labs, I was diagnosed with a perforated intestine. The pill had eroded through my small intestines. Result: ten weeks in the ICU; nothing by mouth; and a weight loss of forty pounds. Trust me; there are easier ways to lose weight!

Not convinced? OK, try this one on for size. After developing diabetes from Agent Orange after a couple of shoot downs in Vietnam, I was placed on a fantastic drug for diabetes, Glucophage (Metformin). I am still on it, by the way. Unfortunately, I developed a kidney stone unrelated to the medicine. To evaluate it, I was given an aptly named kidney dye study. No one knew at the time that Glucophage and the dye used in certain X-ray studies (even CT scans) reacts with Glucophage and forms a substance that shuts down your kidneys. Yes, Tommy Boy, you just won an eight-week stay at ICU Island—complete with dialysis. Whoopee! So, hey, did those episodes really happen to me—a physician? Absolutely. Oh, I know what you're thinking: "You poor bastard. Talk about unlucky!" Well here's the thing. You, too, can easily be a winner in this club. You see, every year, we (well-meaning, well-trained doctors) kill 120,000 patients by medication errors, or ADRs (Adverse Drug Reactions) as they are known in the profession. To put some perspective on that number, that's over twice the number of combat veterans that we lost in all of the Vietnam War. I say again for emphasis and at the risk of boring repetition: "PILLS KILLS."

Now, like a polished politician, I'm going to go back on my words. Some pills and supplements have proven to be really healthy, if not life-changing in a positive sense. But again, my caveat is that, just because of excellent evidence for their efficacy in *some* cases, there is no guarantee that they will be right for *you*. They may interact with meds that you are already taking or your body may just say to you—after downing one or two of these miracles in a pill—"No way, Sweetheart .... And how would you like a nasty case of diarrhea to go with your itchy rash?" *Always* try a supplement or a vitamin/herb one at a time and for two weeks before adding more.

Unfortunately, we have all grown up in a "take-a-pill-for-something society." We are bombarded by commercials pushing new meds on a daily basis. Notice how all of the possible complications are always mentioned (because it's the law) but in a lower voice. I swear. Really listen next time. They always say to "... avoid this product if you are allergic to it or its contents." Really?! Is that a necessary statement? It's like the flight attendant telling me to put on my seatbelt before flying. Come on now. If you don't know that, you shouldn't be allowed to fly. But I digress....

Today there are pills for a cold, the flu, an allergy, a runny nose, sneezing, and on and on and on. Do we really think that a special pill will stop only sneezing but will leave your little nose to run on? Of course not, but the greater the "specialization" and option for products the greater the potential for revenue. Consequently, we become brainwashed into thinking that for each and every ailment or disease there is a specific pill to cure it. No where do you hear "Stop drinking that soda and your allergies, fatigue, joint pain, and a host of other complaints will disappear." Schneider's rule: 'Tis far better to avoid toxins we put into our mouths than to chase the symptoms with a pill (or a supplement, etc.).

That, too, having been said, I admit to taking an eighty-one mg aspirin every night. Why? Because unless you have a medical reason not to take aspirin or an allergic reaction to it, aspirin is virtually life-saving for men and women over fifty years of age. Aspirin has been shown to lower the risk of heart attacks, stroke, and even cancer. Bona fide studies support this? Yes. Sounds good to me.

D-3 is a derivative of vitamin D but not all of us can derive it. Eighty-plus percent of us are deficient in D-3. So what? Well, again, D-3 has been shown to be effectively harmless and protects from cancer, dementia, heart disease, and bone loss. If taken at night and with or after a fatty dinner, it also helps with sleep. By the way, I say "fatty dinner" to mean inclusion of foods like bacon or butter in the meal or any other fat because D (as well as A, E, and K) are fat soluble and, thus, get absorbed into your system in a fatty food environment. I learned the hard way. I once had a patient with very low D-3 and osteoporosis. I put her on D-3 but her levels never went up. Questioning her again, I discovered that a friend told her to take her D-3 on an empty stomach first thing in the morning! Ahhh, what would we do without friends like that? Maybe live longer!

Now how about this crazy fish oil (Omega 3) thing? Healthy, hype, or hoax? Let's put it this way, the only creatures who do *not* need it are … fish. Another source is from a tiny sea animal called krill. (Whales love them!) Omega 3 is a fatty acid used for energy, cell building, brain support, and so much more. The only problem with fish oil is that it is gastric. You can get GI discomfort and heartburn from it. These symptoms usually pass. (What a great pun—right

Steve?). Krill tends to cause fewer problems—especially if you freeze the capsules or use the lemon flavored liquid—as the GI issues are pretty much eliminated. (Oh, there I go again! And to think I never took a single pun-making class!) One more little caveat here. Omega 3 can act as a "blood thinner." That is, bleeding can take longer to stop. So be sure to stop taking it and tell your doctor that you have been using it prior to any scheduled surgery.

B complex (B, B1, B2, B3, B5, B6, B12, and folic acid) and Vitamin C are also strong contenders for our attention … and use. They are great sources for energy and as anti-tox-ins—first rate, in fact. These are best taken in the morning as they may tend to keep you awake. "But, hey, doc, what about multivitamins?" Glad you asked. Nothing supports a daily multivitamin. Sorry. They are simply not the magic pills that they are advertised to be. Nevertheless, if you are pregnant or on a crash diet or fast, follow your doctor's advice and take one on a daily basis for a while if she so recommends. Otherwise, send your multivitamins to the food-depleted countries of the world—along with a check.

Resveratrol is a newbee on the market. Multiple animal studies have shown its efficacy as an anti-oxidant, and in mice studies there has been significant prolongation of life span. Do I take it? No. It's expensive and I already take a plethora of meds and supplements. The positive effect of resveratrol is on a segment of your genes called telomeres. (*Telos* in Greek is "the end" and that's exactly where telomeres sit on your genes.) With aging, our telomeres drop off and this process promotes death. Resveratrol protects your telomeres. Should you take it? This one is really your call. No question that it's one to watch and research. I'm soon to start …maybe…probably.

Not a vitamin but a mineral is magnesium. Unbelievably wonderful and often overlooked, magnesium is the supplement of choice for some cardiac arrhythmias. Shortly after my bypass surgery while in the ICU—which they now call "the Tommy" around here—yet again, I went into an arrhythmia and was immediately given intravenous magnesium. End of problem. Yes, I love magnesium. Taken at night before bedtime, five-hundred mgs will help you to sleep better than a sleeping pill and without the morning grogginess. It also acts as a laxative (hence, Milk of Magnesia). If you develop diarrhea while taking it, simply cut your dose in half. For diabetics, it helps with insulin and gets sugar into your cells. Burning feet? Magnesium is fantastic. Also, it's an amazing muscle relaxant. I never miss a night.

You may have noticed that I have not yet mentioned the Popeye stuff: iron. There now, I have. But only as a no-no. You do need iron, but you get tons of it in whatever your diet is now. Want some fun? Take your cereal—if it says it contains iron—sprinkle some on the table and put a magnet near it. The cereal will move to the magnet. Iron. Unfortunately, too much iron is a cardo toxic. Not a good thing. And after a woman has ceased menses, she will not need it either. Please do not take iron as a supplement unless you have been diagnosed with iron deficiency anemia or low blood count. A physician needs to monitor your levels once you start an iron regimen. Bottom line: Leave the iron (but not the spinach) to Popeye.

CoQ10 is another one that may be new to you. It doesn't receive the publicity of others, but it has been richly studied. CoQ10 works primarily in the mitochondria of cells—the little powerhouse of energy production in each cell. Drugs like statins and certain antacids lower it from your cells. I do take

CoQ10 (also goes by the name of Ubiquinol) just because of the cardiac studies that show its amazing benefits on the heart. Again, I don't take everything in the vitamin dictionary, and I don't take my use as the gold standard. But … when I needed bypass surgery, my cardiac output (how much blood my heart could pump) was 28%. Normal is 40—80%. Needless to say, I was in the proverbial "hurt locker." After the bypass surgery and five subsequent stents, my output went to 62%. It has been twelve years and many hours of pushups and rowing, but my output today is 75%. My cardiologist is astounded and asks, "How?" I say, "CoQ10 and … *row, row, row!*"

Obviously, this topic is a passion of mine and there's simply not enough time and space for me to cover it completely here. But today, there is so much information available on supplements, hormones, and elements that the problem lies in where to find the truth. Sales and revenue stoke the truth fire so that now the subject has become a raging furnace. So, to help you through all of this, I would like to recommend an excellent book on this topic by Dr. Pam Smith. Extremely well versed on this topic, she is also a warrior of truth—the trustworthy kind. Her book is *What You Must Know about Vitamins, Minerals, Herbs and More.* It is published by Square One Publishing.

Now, if I may, a few parting points.

> Take any pill with a full glass of water. More than one pill? OK, small sips and then finish with a full glass of water.

Make sure your doctor knows about all of your "over-the-counters."

Just 'cause it's over-the-counter doesn't mean it's safe.

Talk to your pharmacist about interactions. They are wizards on this very important subject.

Avoid grapefruit juice with or near the taking of your pills.

Get your pills out of the bathroom. Steam/heat decreases their strength by 50% or more.

Unlabeled pill? Looks like something you take? Throw it out! You don't know.

Most pills last way beyond the expiration date printed on the label. Up to two years. But if it's a critical medicine like nitroglycerin or a diabetes med, don't risk it; follow the expiration information.

Main rule: When in doubt, throw it out!

And here's an old maxim for you to ponder (with my tongue only partially in my cheek): "Most doctors know little about disease, less about medicines, and practically nothing about being a patient!"

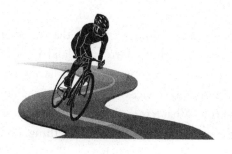

Chapter 7

# Vices: Living (Well) with Our Flaws

First, some ground rules for my writing and your reading this chapter. I am going to do here what I did in Chapters 4 and 5. After I discuss vices in general and mine, specifically, I am going to give Tom a chance to comment to see if I have been fair with, too easy on, or too hard on myself in terms of the medical ramifications of my behavior. Once again, he has no idea that I am going to put him on the spot with this, but I think this approach lends transparency, fun, and, yes, a level of risk to the substance of this chapter. Here we go.

Time for total disclosure ... and some more fun. Lest you think I am one who never crosses the line, I need to set the record straight. Like just about everybody, I have faults—especially when it comes to taking care of myself. I'll cut right to the chase with respect to *diet*: I eat too much salt; I eat processed food; I often eat late (9:00 PM or later); I drink more alcohol than I should; I eat more than my share of pasta, potatoes, and rice (those darn carbs and high glycemics!); and I don't drink enough water. (I will have a few words to say about non-dietary vices later on in this chapter.) So … questions arise. What has made me come to these conclusions regarding my dietary vices? What, if anything, do I intend to do about them? How will my choices affect my dedication to aging deliberately?[27]

Let's start with **the salt issue**.[28] Perhaps you have a salt issue as well. Why do I think that I eat too much salt? First, I may need to remind you that I have hypertension, which, by the way, is controlled beautifully by exercise, meds, and even diet—despite what I view as too much salt and alcohol intake. I *know* that all processed food is full of sodium, but I do try to avoid eating such foods as much as I can. This means that I buy in bulk, not boxes. If it comes in a box or, often, in a can or on a plate at a typical restaurant, it probably has lots of sodium. I *know* that some salt is essential, but anything above the recommended amount of 1500-2300 mg per day is not good. And the more one goes over that recommended amount, the worse it can be. I also consume sodium believing that, since I am over fifty and have hypertension (even though it is under control), I should stay close to the 1500 mg per day

---

[27] I know some of you are thinking that there are some sleep issues here, as well. Fair enough. But I will say that I, most fortunately, have been blessed with the ability to sleep really well virtually every night. If I have a night or two each week where I only get five or six hours, I can tell you it will have been a very restful five or six hours. It is a rare morning when I have trouble rising and shining.

[28] I do know that including a reasonable amount of iodized salt in the diet is a good way to be sure we are getting enough iodine—an element that we need but our bodies do not manufacture. The sodium we take in from processed foods or even sea salt is not helpful here.

limit. The problem is that I estimate my normal sodium intake per day is probably about 2500 mg. I do not eat much in the way of processed foods—except for those darn chips ... you know, the Kettle chips and other types of "healthy" chips that are relatively low in bad fats and calories but still pretty high in sodium. And I am also a lover of salty tomato-y drinks like bloody Mary mix, V-8, and Very Veggie juice.

**Processed Food.** We probably better start out with a definition here. I view processed food as food that has been altered from its natural state in order to make its consumption more convenient and/or flavorful. Processing can be done in a number of ways: additives (e.g., salt, nitrates, nitrites, sugar, fat), dehydration, and freezing are, perhaps, the most common. And ... *not all processed food is bad for us.* It really comes down to *how* the food has been altered and *for what purpose.* Let's start with fresh-frozen fruit and veggies. If the freezing process adds virtually nothing to the food, the produce may actually end up being more nutritious for us than so-called fresh food found at the grocery store. The problem is that much of the processed food that we eat—either from the grocery store or when we eat at a restaurant—contains unhealthy additives. And—here is where my processed food vice comes in—I eat my share of salsas, chips and crackers, and processed meats. (Yes, even the "uncured" turkey bacon that I so enjoy does go through a modified curing process, is processed, and is not, by any stretch of the imagination, health food.) So ... what am I doing about this vice? Simply stated, I am trying to keep it under control/in moderation/*balanced.* In fact, very recently, I have begun to cut back on the processed meat (the turkey bacon and chicken sausage) I am so fond of enjoying for breakfast. I also try to eat the chips and crackers with the least fat, salt, and other bad stuff while keeping my intake to a modest amount (even on holidays never more than about three hundred calories per day). I give myself lots of tests (e,g., almost daily blood pressure checks, a close eye on what my bathroom scale shows when I hop on every couple of days, my waistline, and semi-annual cholesterol checks) to be sure that I am not losing ground. I have been balancing all of my eating and drinking vices with a good blend of other healthy, highly nutritional foods, supplements, and exercise in this manner for about fifteen years now and ... and so far, so good. Like Tom says, the key to lots of this is "WHOA, not NO!"

**Eating late.** My fairly regular late evening dining experiences began at least twenty years ago when I started teaching night courses at colleges and universities near my duty stations while I was in the Navy. I will note here that teaching is extraordinarily energizing and healthy for me. Many were the evenings that I would drive to my evening class—often starting around six and sometimes going until after 10:00 PM—already bushed from an exhausting day as a Navy lawyer, almost ready to fall asleep at the wheel. And, after hours of the mental and physical challenges of teaching freshman composition or an American literature survey class, I would head home—invigorated and fully charged. My point here is that by the time I drove home, calmed down a bit, and, yes, had a glass of wine while preparing dinner, it was often 11:00 before I sat down to eat. This kind of a day was not my everyday routine, mind you. But there have been many weeks when it would be at least a three-day experience each week.[29] I am now retired and am not even teaching one class at the moment,

---

[29] Usually an evening class on Tuesday, Wednesday, and Thursday nights.

so there is no scheduling reason for me to have to eat later than the average American diner. Nevertheless, I rarely take my first bite of din-din until at least seven o'clock—a compromise with Barbara who normally prefers an earlier dinner time. You see, I really enjoy cooking and eating, and I look at dinner as the highlight of what I have tried to make a productive and fun day. Consequently, it makes perfect sense to me, I believe, to have (and savor) a long dinner hour as close to the end of my day as possible (note, I did not say "reasonable").

Now, along with my dinner hour (or two), during which I prepare a full, well-balanced[30] meal virtually every night, comes eating/dining vice number three: **too much alcohol.** Having a drink during dinner preparations and wine with dinner is customary for me. Note that I am including this as a *vice*, not a recommendation. The problem is that a shot of booze and a glass of wine every night of the week amounts to fourteen drinks per week and, according to every account I have read that goes beyond moderate (i.e., *balanced*) alcohol consumption and into the realm of heavy drinking. You see, you don't have to be an alcoholic to be classified as a heavy, unhealthy, or problem drinker. The fact that folks who are heavy drinkers may be perfectly civil when imbibing and may seem to be generally quite healthy is misleading. Heavy drinking is just plain hard on our bodies—especially key organs, our cognitive ability, and our sleep. And of course there is the ever

---

[30] Each night I try to prepare and enjoy a dinner that consists of reasonable amounts of salad (as much cabbage, onions, carrots, kale, and tomatoes as possible), a protein (usually chicken, fish, turkey, or beans), a starch (often a potato, some brown rice, quinoa, or couscous), and a lightly steamed or sautéed vegetable (broccoli, asparagus, squash, and zucchini are real favorites). Desserts are simply not in the mix—although I am slowly attempting to start having a small piece of dark chocolate to finish meal on occasion. Doctor Tom's orders!

present issue of collateral damage from intoxication which can result from falling and doing stupid stuff like breaking a favorite antique, misplacing things, or, heaven forbid, climbing into a car and creating any sort of mayhem. I am attempting to make a point here—for you and for me—without appearing to preach. Let's face it; for most of us, drinking is a true pleasure of life, a fun way to enjoy friends or a wonderful meal. But, left unchecked and out of balance, it also can do serious harm and is certainly not conducive to aging deliberately and, in extreme cases, is not conducive to aging ... period. Please enjoy your alcoholic drinks, if you like—but, as the excellent conventional wisdom dictates, in moderation.[31]

**Non-dietary vices.** The potential here is huge and a lot of this is attitudinal. I will leave it to you to determine the degree of evil or naughtiness associated with each of these. Some of the most common and most obvious ones that come to mind are greed, unchecked profanity,[32] lying, stealing, smoking (and virtually any use of any tobacco product), cruelty to and/or unjustifiably harming human and non-human animals (lots of room for subjectivity here), wastefulness, selfishness,

---

[31] I do not make this final point glibly. "Moderation" may be relatively easy to understand when a person is sober. But drinking goes straight to the part of the brain that controls reason and judgment. Consequently, even a couple of drinks can have a measureable impact on our self-control, and knowing when to say "when" may not be as easy as it may seem. I suggest setting limits and staying within them—especially when driving may be required.

[32] I am not against letting out virtually every profane utterance I choose—when the time and circumstances are appropriate. In fact, I think using the F-Bomb, for example, can be wonderful for de-stressing and is often even a good source for humor. Discretion and, once again, balance can keep swearing and those of us who choose to use such expressions a pretty harmless vice. Overuse, I think we can all agree, is boring at best and really obnoxious, crude, and downright antisocial at worst. As is the case with just about every component of aging deliberately, balanced use works; abuse does not.

stubbornness, mean spiritedness …. Obviously, some of these are no-brainers and have no place in the life of anyone who is attempting to age deliberately. But there is one (drug use—any form of tobacco, use of illegal drugs, and misuse of prescription drugs) that I want to discuss separately from all the rest and will save for the end of the chapter, and there are at least two others that come to mind that are not so easy to evaluate: gambling and sun exposure.

Let's start with **gambling**. Fact is I know some very deliberate agers who *do* gamble. The key for them, however, is that they do their gambling—weather it comes in the form of lottery tickets or an evening at a casino or a night of poker with their card group—in a controlled, *balanced* manner. They have a realistic limit on what they can afford to lose in a given session. Gambling for these folks is truly entertainment, fun; it is not an obsession or a way for them to try to make some needed extra money. Whether it's gambling or virtually anything else in life—whether it is an activity that is normally considered to be a vice or not—if something has hold of a person and that person plans his/her life's activities around that activity, there is something wrong. When a person is distracted to the point of losing balance, concentrating *on* balance is impossible. And, without balance, there can be no deliberateness in *any*thing—especially aging.

That gets us to **sun exposure**. I am going to go out on a limb and say that the sun is *not* an enemy to good health. We need to get our fair share of it to remain healthy. Once again, the need for *balance* when it comes to our exposure to the sun is incredibly important. I learned my lesson following my three-year tour of duty in Hawaii. In addition to a pretty full work and teaching schedule, I managed to take full advantage of the beautiful Hawaiian weather which meant lots of time on and under the water and running three to eight miles each day along with the occasional ten K or half marathon race. A full and healthy lifestyle you may be thinking, but the problem was that most of my time in the sun was with little to no sun screen and no shirt. I usually sported only a ball cap and running shorts (and running shoes and socks if I was not doing time on the boat). I never once had a sun burn, but I was doing damage to my skin on virtually a daily basis. About eight months after I had left Hawaii for my new duty station in Pensacola, Florida …. You guessed it—skin cancer, lesions on my right temple and over my front right collar bone. The surgery was successful but the point was made. Now it's broad-brimmed hats, plenty of sun screen, and no bare, shirtless stuff except for time in the water.

Now, some thoughts on **drugs**. Tobacco products are bad news and you know it. The evidence is in and it all points to choosing total abstention or choosing to add unnecessary and probable life-threatening risks to you and even those around you in the case of smoking. Any other choice is unwise and unhealthy. Easy for me to say because I don't smoke; I know. But I used to smoke cigarettes and cigars and I even chewed tobacco (perhaps the most addicting from of tobacco use), but I quit. If you use tobacco, please use every resource that you can to kick the habit or, more accurately, the addiction. Next, I may throw you a bit with what I am about to say about illegal drugs—especially their sale. I'll get right to the point: After giving the matter years of thought, I now think that—subject to controls regarding sales to minors, use by public servants, and regulations involving use while operating vehicles, etc.—all sale of virtually any drug should be decriminalized. Prohibition (of alcohol) did not work and made millionaires out of criminals, and the same has happened with respect to the current drug scene and the "war on drugs" that we, as a society, have been fighting (and losing) for decades now. I am certainly *not* advocating unhealthy drug abuse, of course, but I do think the medical evidence points to some substances such as cannabis as having definite positive effects on some folks with certain medical conditions when used with moderation. That brings us to (currently) legal prescription drugs that can and often are abused. There really is not much to be said here: Abuse is abuse. If the prescription says one pill per day and the person chooses to take two or more, this is abuse and it is unhealthy—period. I think Tom would add that, since many physicians prescribe so many medications without getting to the root of the *need* for them, the very issuance of the prescription for a condition that could be corrected by, say, more exercise, a change in diet, or both is a way of creating drug abuse situations. I know that he will have much more to say about this in his section of this chapter.

By the way, and finally, I think another vice is being preachy. So I am going to wind down my take on vices now. It isn't easy to discuss vices and their impact on a healthy, fulfilling, deliberately-lived life without seeming to be shaking a finger in other people's faces—especially when I admit to having my share of experience with almost every vice that I have discussed here. So, I will close my part of this chapter now with the thought that I know we, with our great human capacity for making mistakes, will, indeed, make mistakes and do stupid stuff once in a while. Forgive yourself when you slip up and don't be afraid to apologize to others affected by your gaffs. Just try not to make apologizing for your behavior an everyday part of your life.

The ball's in your court, Tom.

When I was a young boy, I was steeped in Catholicism. I hated Saturdays because we would all go to "confession" and tell the priest our "sins" of the week. My sin was always the same: "impure thoughts" about Christiana Fitzgerald—the beauty of the sixth grade. I really grew to detest "confession." So why is it that, at 70+ years old, I now have the same feeling in my gut? Oh yeah, that's right! Steve has me writing about vices. Will it ever end?!

OK, OK, as much as it hurts, I'll venture into the realm of personal vices as they relate to healthy aging. Now, I have just finished reading Steve's "mea culpa" (sorry, old church Latin for "my fault") and I am again seriously annoyed. Worse than the confessional. But please read his section again because it is spot on.

I, too, am a salt-a-holic. My addiction comes in the form of tomato or V-8 juice. I've cut back to just twice a week, but it's tough. What's that you say? They make a low-sodium version? Been there, done that and needed to add salt to not waste the bottle. Go real or go home! That's my motto! Now, unlike Steve, I don't have hypertension but too much salt is just plain toxic for all of us. And make no mistake; it's in all of our shelved and processed foods. That said, I'll confess a little more: Through a Meryl Streep movie, I will tub out on popcorn for sure. I always ask for broccoli at the concession counter and dutifully turn to my wife sheepishly reporting that they don't have any. Gotta go with popcorn. Remember: Go real or go home. I love Steve's guide of 1500 mgs of salt per day, but there's a problem. I usually don't keep my salt scale with me. (No, I really don't own one.) So what can we do?

Great advice from Steve: Weigh yourself. Keep close tabs on your scale. If you notice a sudden increase in poundage while your basic calorie intake has remained stable, you can be pretty sure what the culprit is. It's water being retained by excess salt intake. This happens more often than you may think. You can use green tea or even an herbal diuretic (water remover) to respond. Just don't do so for more than a week because in losing sodium (salt) you will also lose potassium and you need that desperately to maintain heart stabilization and to avoid cramps and high blood pressure.

I won't bore you here by reiterating Steve's salient points. They are all really fantastic and very much worth paying attention to. But, if I may, I'd like to add some personal thoughts on how I try to manage my booboos. Eating late is my toughie. Even if I finish eating dinner at a relatively early hour, late-night snacking hits me like "Jaws," the great white shark. And here's the thing: I know it, and yet I still do it. It all comes down to that nasty word *change*. I'm convinced that change is just the hardest thing we can ever do in any endeavor in our lives. So change for me comes in baby steps. Tonight, I'll feel the good feeling of fullness by having a soda water with a splash of fruit juice in it. Still not working for me? I'll try adding slow, small bites of natural peanut butter. Friday? I'm all in for garlic bread. Sorry. One of my favorite sane snacks at night is sprinkled shaved parmesan cheese over parchment cooking paper (find it next to aluminum foil at the grocery store) … and microwave it for about forty-five seconds. It comes out like a Cheetos pancake and with a tad bit of salsa … yum, yum! The point, of course, is to make small changes and know that you are gonna stumble once in a while. I love stumble nights. But no fair doing two stumble nights in a row.

Yes, Steve, I am a huge fan of dark chocolate and I'm delighted that you're converting. Sooo good and less of a rise in blood sugar and insulin than if you ate a banana. That's right. Bananas are loaded with fructose and it bypasses a host of biochemistry and goes directly into the blood stream. Remember the caution on "high fructose corn syrup" in, for example, soda? Now, I'm a non-alcohol drinker and so I must add that one drink a day is probably great. But think of it as a glass of pure white sugar. Still, OK, but two, three, or more … Don't even try to tell me that you're on a diet or that you want to lose weight. Ain't happening, my friend.

Recreational drugs? Not a fan and definitely not a user. Many are addicting and (with the important exception of medicinal uses of marijuana, for example) not a good practice for those of us who are interested in good health and longevity. That said, we spend billions and billions of dollars on incarceration of prisoners here in the United States. We have more prisoners than any ten countries combined. And 65% are confined for the use of "illegal" drugs. The question of legalizing all drugs, with guidelines, would never make it as a question on "Jeopardy." In my state, as an example, we have an eighteen-year-old African American man in prison for thirteen years. He was arrested with fifteen ounces of marijuana. Are you kidding me?! Bottom line: Steve and I are in complete agreement on this one. Gosh, I hate agreeing with him … again!

When I think about this chapter on vices, I'm reminded of my favorite bromide. Trite, yes, but oh so true for me. Here goes: "In the end, only Kindness matters." How fitting for each of us. And, by the way, that Kindness deal applies first and foremost to ourselves. What a great thought to start each day. So go ahead, Steve. Keep up your strong desire to reach out with humor, good will, and a passion for excellent health and … have another square of rich dark chocolate. Enjoy, my good friend.

One final thought: "Too much of a good thing … is just that."

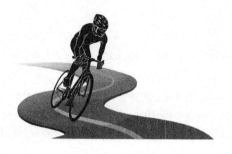

# Chapter 8

# *Appearance and the Four of Each of Us*

Let me be perfectly clear about the subject of this title: I am talking about *physical* appearance. Consequently, while brief, this chapter may be one of the more provocative ones in the book—if not *the* most provocative. At the heart of the matter is this question: Why should we think it is important to look good, to make a pleasing appearance especially when we are out and about? Stated another way, why should it matter what others think of the way we present ourselves— physically? I think the answer to these questions lies in who we regard as the most important observer of how we look: others ... or ourselves.

First, I need to clarify a couple of things. Most important is that by *physical appearance* I am focusing on grooming, being well kempt, hygiene, looking (and being) healthy, being quick with a smile; you know ... things that are outward manifestations of the best of who we really are inside who we *really* are. (No typo there. I meant that exactly the way I wrote it. Make sense ...?) I am *not* talking about accoutrements like designer clothing, expensive jewelry, the latest styles, high-end sports cars, and other things that are more of a reflection of finances and self-indulgence than living and aging deliberately in the Thoreauesque meaning of the term. Nor am I advocating for the other end of the spectrum occupied by our T-shirt wearing friend I spoke of earlier—who, by the way, obviously had not had a shave recently, had not bothered to wear clean clothes, was quite overweight, and was simply not going to be bothered ... with just about anything, apparently. After all, why *should* he be?

Being healthy—emotionally and physically—is something that we should celebrate ... openly. And I believe we do this or can do this or should do this because we love ourselves. In other words, we look our best because we want to do this for *ourselves*. It is not or should not, in my view, be a means to try to either impress others by adorning ourselves in the spoils of our success or by making a point to look our worst as a statement of misplaced independence or individuality which tends simply to drive others away. And with these opening comments I think I have already arrived at the controversial component of this chapter. Some good questions may already be forming in your mind. What is the harm in wearing your favorite (and expensive) jewels when going out on the town or treating yourself to owning and driving an expensive sports car on the one hand? Or, on the other, why should a person be regarded as simply not caring about appearance if his clothes are ill-fitting or he is a bit or very scruffy? After all, looking presentable takes effort and has a cost.

And this leads us to yet another aspect of concern for appearance: nips, tucks, and other assists from doctors and others interested in promoting physical beauty or making a statement. First of all, please remember that my emphasis is on doing our best with what we have—not necessarily to look beautiful or handsome but rather to look our unadulterated best. Remember: This is about *you* not others' perceptions of you. That said, I am not about to wage war on the considered decisions of some to have a relatively low invasive procedure done to improve a physical blemish that may be bothersome to the person contemplating the procedure—a procedure like eye lid surgery that may serve to improve a person's eye sight as well as his/her perception of their appearance. Aren't very acceptable practices of reasonable ear piercings and tattoos, for example, quite the norm these days? Ahh, but what is "reasonable?" Herein lies the rub. What I think is or is not "reasonable" is not at issue here. The *reason* for the physical alteration and the degree of balance involved *are* at issue.

Let's consider a couple of relatively typical examples. First, let's consider the thirty-something married woman who is not particularly well endowed and whose husband is quite persistent in stating his desires that she undergo a breast enhancement procedure, OK … a boob job. She finally gives in and has the procedure which turns out as well as it could. In this case, she is relatively ambivalent, personally, about the "improvement," but her husband is delighted. In the second scenario, we have a middle-aged man in a committed non-marital relationship[33] who has always wanted (for reasons that are of no particular importance here) to have a raging skull tattooed on

---

[33] I am consciously developing scenarios in which the key parties are in important relationships in order to increase the personal dynamics of their choices.

the side of his neck. His partner is not happy about this and has been quite vocal in his objections with this concept. The man gets the tattoo anyway and is quite satisfied with how it looks. Both relationships endure—despite the personal feelings of each of the parties. I think you probably know where I am going with this: Selflessness vs. selfishness—neither is necessarily a good thing, but how do they differ from healthy self-expression, which is. Yes, you guessed it; the answer is *balance.* In the cases of the breast enhancement and very obvious tattoos that I described above, balance, for a number of reasons, is lacking. I have stronger negative feelings about the man who would pressure his wife into having a surgical procedure that she does not really want and her apparent lack of the sufficient self-esteem to deny his wishes than I do with the neck tattoo guy. Yet, in both cases, there definitely appears to be an issue with the Self of at least three of the folks in the scenarios.

Let's take a look at this physical appearance thing as it relates to balance from yet another perspective: Madison Avenue. Specifically, it seems that we have been told for decades now that thin or down-right skinny (especially for women) is sexy and cool and desirable. Being "full-figured" or heavy or plump or—you choose a term—is something to be avoided if a woman is to be regarded as desirable. There is normally very little discussion about nutrition or exercise as entire industries compete to sell "skinny" with clothing, supplements, "diets," and all the rest. During the last ten years or so, however, there has been a growing movement that has been pushing back against the thin-is-beautiful movement. "Full-figured" models—pitching everything from clothing to hair color to vacation destinations—are now seen by many as providing a much-needed alternative to the concepts of physical attractiveness that has prevailed for over fifty years in most Western cultures. And so the battle lines between big is beautiful and skinny is sexy have been drawn between those who are regarded—usually unscientifically—as over or under weight.[34]

I recently listened to an interview with Melissa McCarthy who is currently very popular in movies, in social media, on television (including talk shows), in magazines, and just about everywhere else. As you probably know despite having lost a considerable amount of weight, she is still obese—not by my or anyone else's subjective standards, but clinically. Melissa does not seem to be concerned about her current size; in fact, she celebrates it. While she is no longer morbidly obese, she seems to be content to remain heavy. She exudes self-confidence, contentment, and pride in every part of her appearance. After all, doing so endears her to a significant percentage of Americans. In fact, Melissa is certainly not alone in how she feels about the topic of beauty relative to girth. Moreover, she stands as the perfect contrast to many models, film and music stars, and others who have been held up to epitomize attractiveness, sexiness, and beauty mainly because of their far less corpulent bodies. And, in the meantime, Melissa is making a fortune because she is regarded by many as funny, entertaining, and a good role model for those dealing with weight and, consequently, self-esteem issues. I get it.

What I also get is that just about everyone involved in

---

[34] Of course, such terms do suggest a strong degree of subjectivity since what certain cultures or specific individuals may regard as over or under weight will differ rather dramatically. Therefore, it will be very helpful to this discussion if we can agree that nutritionists and other healthcare experts state that there are certain accepted parameters for weight and body fat percentages that can be used to gauge what weights are truly healthy for a person based on key factors like sex, height, and frame type, for example.

the debate that I have just outlined is missing the point: *being clinically too thin or too heavy is a wellness issue.* I just want to reach out to folks and make the point that balance is as much at the heart of weight and physical attractiveness as it is with everything else. Feeling good about who we are is a truly wonderful thing, but if we base that feeling on how we think we look in the eyes of *others*—using weight or clothing or the cars we drive—we are deceiving ourselves profoundly. I really like what Ms. McCarthy has done to point out the folly of the perception that the only way a woman can be desirable is for her to have a figure like Barbie. But I profoundly disagree with her that being as big as you feel like being is a good thing because it simply is not physically healthy and, I would argue, neither is she.

I am keenly aware that some of you may not be nodding your heads in agreement with me at this point, and that is perfectly fine with me. I feel that a discussion like this is absolutely essential, however, if we are to reach any sort of common ground on the relationship between physical appearance—in all of its forms—and balance, health, and aging deliberately. As you have seen so far and will continue to be evident throughout this book, Tom and I are firmly convinced that aging well and maintaining quality lives and longevity simultaneously is a matter of paying attention to just about everything while having a really good time doing so.

This gets us to the sub-title of this chapter: "The Four of Each of Us." You see, I have a theory about those of us who make some effort to be at least minimally mindful of our relationships to ourselves—those whom we know and those whom we do not know or know only in a certain social context. My theory is based on the notion that socially conscious/

aware people from, say, late childhood or early adolescence and older are actually four people with respect to their relationships with others in a social order. First, there is the person who I am when I am completely by myself—no one else around to offend or impress or engage with in any way. This is the time for intimate and intense personal grooming, uninhibited flatulence, nose picking, singing loudly and out of key, and all the other stuff we should be perfectly happy doing *when we are alone*—pretty much no holds barred in terms of non-destructive/non-violent personal behavior.

The second person is the person I am when I am around my most intimate friends and family members. I am very close to and comfortable with these folks and know they will appreciate and understand and certainly not judge just about anything that I say and/or do—once again, barring destructive or violent behavior. I fundamentally believe that we all need these close folks—just as much as we need time to be completely alone every so often—and we are better off by having such people in our lives. We don't need lots of these friends and/or family members. Just a few will do, but oh how important they are!

Then we have person number three. This is the person I am when I am simply out and about and am doing whatever I need to do in society/civilization to get things done. This person number three is extraordinarily important and, I believe, is a good barometer for how balanced we are in terms of our social selves. This is the person who is challenged to behave in a civil manner when others whom he/she may not know are not. Driving comes to mind. If someone does something that is not very smart or possibly dangerous in the car in front or in back of me, do I deal with the bad behavior by being diligent and possibly even understanding in my response? Or do I lash out, flip the person the bird, or react in any number of ways, thus taking the chance of significantly escalating the situation? A host of other questions about this sort of situational, person-number-three behavior come to mind: Do I hold a door open for a stranger as we enter a store together? Am I quick with a smile? Do I bother to put on a pair of clean casual slacks and bother to comb my hair (if I have any) when I head to the mall to buy a new toaster? Do I project a positive, healthy attitude about life in general? Is Chapter 1 coming to mind right now?

And, finally, there is person number four. This is who I am when I am in my most polished social role. This is how I act when I am interviewing for a new job or when I am in the company of someone for whom I have the highest level of respect—say, my best friend's mother or some great humanitarian. This is not to say that virtually all animals—human and non-human alike—don't deserve our respect. I am just saying that there are some occasions when we want and need to be especially solicitous.

So there you have it: The four of each of us. But there is still more to be said about this. Specifically, we need to consider yet another question. Specifically, how do we grow to gain and practice a sense of civility and decorum without losing our connection with the very essence of who we really are? In other words, how do we grow up but still maintain that incredibly important contact with who we are when we are born or as young children—before all of the socializing and conforming that parents, teachers, friends, and many other mostly well-intentioned beings and entities lay on us. How do we remain true to who we really are and still play and work well with others? I think the answer, once again, is *Balance*. My partner, Barbara, says that I am a goofball. And she loves that goofiness about me; as do I. You see, while I believe that I *am* civil and well-adjusted and mindful of what should and should not be done in various social settings, I have grown *up* with age ... not old with it. I have not forgotten how (and *when*) to be childlike or downright silly and when it is perfectly OK if not required to reach down to the unfiltered me and let it out. This ability has taken me some years to develop and I didn't even realize that it mattered until I was in my forties. So now I think I get it: How to balance social responsibility, civility, and responsible adult behavior with the need to remember who I was as a child and how I really am at the core and to be unafraid to reach down and rely on that core-Steve when I need to make really tough choices or to be creative or to give those closest to me my most profound love. In other words, the goal is to be in person number four mode in most social situations but to be informed and guided by my most essential and unaffected Self. As I suggested earlier, this has not always been easy for me but I am getting the hang of it and it feels really good!

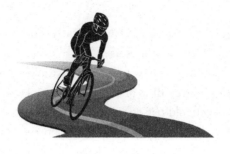

Chapter 9

# Quirkiness: A Little Goes a Long Way

This seems like a good time to take a closer look at behavior. And here I am addressing behavior that may seem relatively inconsequential to the actor but which can be irritating if not downright repulsive to those who endure it. These are things that I have noticed being done by others (and, on occasion, by me). Most are not necessarily critical to aging in a physically healthy manner. In fact, they are far more idiosyncratic and quirky than they are health-related. This business is, however, fundamental to aging well, deliberately, in a general sense. In any case, the subject is certainly worth our attention and may lead to an "ahh-haa" moment or two and even some laughs.

## Moaning, Groaning, and Other Totally Unnecessary (and Annoying) "Old-Person Noises"

Have you ever noticed how folks who have allowed themselves to become old—regardless of their age in actual years—tend to make what I call "old-person" noises? As the title of this sub-section suggests, I am referring to all that blubbering … moaning, groaning, grunting, snorting, hacking, incessant and unnecessary throat clearing and coughing, thinking out loud, and, oh yes, belching and farting. Hey, don't get me wrong here; I completely understand *occasional* utterances of relief or exhaustion or an *occasional* self-pitying moan or groan when one is feeling sore or sick. I celebrate the release of all the methane one wishes to let loose of in the privacy of one's own company. And I am a proponent of good, healthy conversations with ourselves (when we are really *by ourselves*). I also understand that we all should be allowed a little lee-way here. Some things just sneak out no matter how hard we try to stay in control.

My gripe here is with the folks who simply don't care how irritating and obnoxious their cacophony of annoying noises and utterances may be to others and who often let them fly knowing full well how downright distasteful and nasty they are to those around them. It is really a lot like what young children often do out of ignorance or to be silly or annoying. This behavior is symptomatic of those old fuddy-duddies who espouse the belief that it is acceptable and even enviable to grow old but not to grow *up*. As you know by now, this is exactly the opposite of what I believe that aging deliberately is about. So, if we can exert some control over such things, let's just do it. Those around us will really appreciate it.[35]

---

[35] While we are at it, nose/ear picking, pimple popping, butt scratching, and other hands-on personal "grooming" practices—all perfectly OK and even

## The Inattentive "Huh/What?" and Interruptions[36]

I can't tell you how many times I have been around couples who simply don't communicate effectively on a regular basis. Sorry, gentlemen, but my anecdotal observations over the past sixty years or so, lead me to conclude that men are more guilty of certain miscommunication practices than women are. Think about it. How many times have you been around a traditional married couple (more often than not, a pair that has been together for a long time) and listened to them as they "talk" during a trip in the car or at breakfast or at the grocery store? One of them (usually the woman) will say something that the other is certainly very capable of hearing, and the response to the initial point or question is "Huh?" or "What?" or some other "response" indicating lack of interest, attention, or agreement which always requires needless repetition of what was said in the first place. Later on I will say a little more about patience, but requiring a person to constantly repeat what is clearly discernible calls for something beyond ordinary patience and, if you are a practitioner of this inattentive and inconsiderate behavior, please consider some behavior modification. Sooner or later someone's "patience" is going to run out, and your life may be in jeopardy!

Just last week I had to conduct a little informal business with a couple in their mid-sixties. I have known them casually for about fifteen years, and they have been married for at least twice that long. During the fifteen minutes that I was in their company, they interrupted each other—again, the man was

necessary at times … while in the bathroom or some other private space—are also usually looked upon with varying levels of disgust by most reasonable people when such activities are conducted in public. I touched on this earlier in Chapter 8 when I talked about "The Four of Each of Us."

[36] This one is especially important for partners.

the more egregious offender—repeatedly. And I became quite confused as to what they—as a couple—really wanted to do about the matter at hand. It was a very simple matter, really, but their inattention and the consequential chaos that resulted was, once again, food for thought. It got me wondering how in the world they and a number of other couples whom I have known could raise children and manage a home together when there was so little effective communication going on. Maybe they have developed a sixth sense or something when they conduct life's business together, but all that I can tell you is that I walked away from our time together with lots of confusion and a headache. This was by no means an isolated experience for me—around this couple or others who have been with each other for more than a few years.

Barbara and others close to me have told me that I am a good listener, a strong communicator. I think that I am and I am proud of this. But I will say that listening—carefully and without interrupting—and responding thoughtfully to others (especially those closest to us) takes effort. I think we all can understand that. Nevertheless, for some reason, many of us either fail to remember the importance of that effort or simply don't care anymore at a certain point as we add years. The results are irritating at best and can often lead to unnecessary confusion, mistakes, and unpleasantness. I, for one, have promised myself to stay in the (communication) game, to pay attention, and to respond in the same way that I have chosen to age—*deliberately*.

### Gratuitous Worrying

I know folks from high-school days and even longer who used to be really good at taking things in stride. I am not talking about the devil-may-care, reckless, or even self-destructive be-havior that hormone riddled high-schoolers often embrace. I am referring to a more mellow, it's-not-that-bad-we-can-prob-ably-work-this-problem-out sort of attitude. Inherent in this is a healthy touch of optimism, a positive spirit, and a realization that things really could be a lot worse. For some of these in-dividuals, normal everyday issues have begun to take on far more significance than before. "Things really aren't all that great" and "What-am-I going-to-do-now(?!)" seem to be the main themes of the day—most days—for some folks. And, all too often, what they are feeling and thinking is manifested by what they do and say without their even realizing it. I could choose to find this behavior quite weird if not a bit frighten-ing, but I choose to see a bit of humor in it—not laughing at the person but more at the folly of the outlook. If you think about it, I'll bet you know exactly what I am talking about here: the gratuitous worrying (often acted out) about things of very little consequence (e.g., finding exactly the right parking place at the grocery store, being less than ten minutes *early* for some appointment, saggy pants on some adolescent (who has a lot more in common with the worrier than they would ever imagine), life-or-death decisions regarding the what and when of dinner tonight, and on and on.

I think this behavior is the product of a number of things: too much free time, fear, incapacity mainly due to physical limitations, impatience, intolerance, anger about "getting old," and other factors that the worriers feel (incorrectly, I believe) that they have no control over. Obviously, attitude is key here. But I believe this worrying/negative attitude can be improved, made more positive. Refocusing on what is good about life and what can be done—within reason—in a positive, productive way to improve what is not good is really important here, and such constructive behavior is not beyond the reach of most folks. Those of us who are not gratuitous worriers can take it upon ourselves to show them the way—tactfully, subtly, by examples that are good for us and (in time) good for the worriers. Perhaps we all could benefit by having another good look at Chapter 1.

## The Good Old Days

Closely related to gratuitous worrying is the incessant longing for "the good old days"—you know ... when the music was better, everyone was nicer, the world was more peaceful, our generation was cooler and did just about everything better, and all the rest of it. Hogwash!! It's the same sort of generational warfare that has been going on for centuries ... and much longer. Our parents bemoaned the same baseless longing and we rolled our eyes (justifiably) at that kind of nonsense the same way many younger folks do when they hear this nonsense today. The fact of the matter is that "things," in general, are not much worse or better than they used to be—twenty, thirty, forty, or two hundred years ago.[37] But they are certainly *different*. And different is often regarded as scary or threatening by folks of any age—especially, however, as they get old.

You know, this good-old-days business is really based to a

---

[37] The one "thing"—and it is a really big one—that is certainly worse than it was a generation and more ago is the overall condition of the environment. By now, there should be no doubt in anyone's mind that climate change, pollution, annihilation of all kinds of non-human animals and flora, and other negative environmental changes have occurred on a huge scale with efforts to enact the sorts of regulations necessary to make real, lasting improvements consistently blocked by those driven by fear, ignorance, and/or greed. On the other hand, equality for people of color, women, and gay folks has made some significant headway over the last fifty years.

large extent on the tendency for most human beings to resist change—especially when change could alter a seemingly relatively comfortable and secure existence. It follows, then that the older we get and, if all has gone pretty well for us in our lives, the more settled we are in our surroundings, the more we want to hang on to what makes us feel comfortable and safe. Sometimes, however, we need to look beyond ourselves a bit. I have a really good example for you. Today is Friday, 26 June 2015. The date may be easily recognizable for some; it may be a date that, along with the Japanese attack on Pearl Harbor, will go down in infamy; or, for me and millions of other Americans, it is one of the truly great days of this generation. Today, the Supreme Court of the United States—in a five-to-four decision—announced its opinion making same-sex marriage legal throughout the land ... *immediately*. It is also interesting to note that yesterday the Supremes—once again in a five-to-four—decision validated an extraordinarily important provision of the Patient Protection and Affordable Care Act (aka "ObamaCare"), helping to further entrench this landmark but highly controversial legislation into the fabric of our society. In addition, this past week saw the Confederate battle flag's removal from government buildings in several southern states.[38] All in all, the past week has been a wondrous

---

[38] This flag has, of course, been a source of controversy for many years. I realize that a few comments here cannot do justice to the complexities of the issue. Let me just say this. On one hand, it has been a symbol of independence and the uniqueness of the American South generating both pride and honor. On the other hand, it recalls the tragedy of the Civil War, the horrors of slavery, and lingering racism. In any case, the decision to remove the flag from positions of honor on government buildings was given a huge push forward by an act of unspeakable violence. The horror of the act is palpable; the irony of what has transpired is overwhelming; the good that can come from tragedy and change is liberating.

time for Progressives; for conservative folks not terribly receptive to change ... not so much. Look, I'm not a change-for-change-sake kind of person. I think logical, strong arguments can be made against many changes in the legal, social, cultural make-up of the United States and many other countries. American public school curricula deleting such courses as band, art, and even foreign languages and increased, almost non-stop testing and mind-numbing administrative responsibilities placed on teachers who just want to teach come to mind. And what about the ubiquitous presence of personal communication devices and the invasion of social networking into every aspect of our lives as a couple of things we may need to think about in this regard? And as long as we are on the subject of change that may not really be for the best, the apparent permanence of the designated hitter in the American League is *really* scary!

The good old days simply never were—except perhaps for a small minority of affluent, straight, white ("preferably" not from Eastern Europe or, heaven forbid, Ireland) men. Romanticizing about a "better" time from our past is not helpful. Working with what we have now and *using the lessons we should have learned from our past and the mistakes we made in that past*[39] to help the world move *forward* is what we who have had the privilege of long life should have as our focus. To me, it's that looking and actually moving forward in a *positive, new* direction—a direction that embraces intelligent, rational, helpful *change*—that really matters. That's where I am and that

---

[39] For example, the near annihilation of native Americans, slavery, Jim Crow, the war in Southeast Asia, a failed war on drugs, corporate greed, the mess in the Middle East begun largely due to a jingoistic, in fact horrific series of foreign policy decisions, wholescale polluting of our environment, intolerance in general, and many more.

is yet another reason why I am happy, healthy, and optimistic as I age deliberately.

## Chronic Indecision

We have all seen it: folks—more often than not, older folks—holding up the works because they simply can't make a decision. It can be one person, a couple, or a group. As recently as yesterday, I saw a couple—in their late sixties—whom I know at the grocery store. Their shopping cart was parked right in the middle of the aisle, and there they stood deliberating out loud about the virtues of one brand of potato chips over another and the cost difference of about six cents per bag. A small traffic jam was forming, so I gave them a friendly "Hello," a big smile, and a courteous "excuse me" as I moved their cart out of the way, thus allowing traffic to pass while they continued their debate. By the way, these folks do not have any unusual physical or mental issues and are quite well off financially. I couldn't help thinking as I moved on: "Get on with your lives, folks!" Yes, I admit that I was being a bit judgmental with this pair; in fact, a reasonable person could argue that this entire chapter is tainted with more than an insubstantial amount of judging. Fair enough, but I see it all as an informed open, candid discussion about things that we should pay attention to—especially as we age. Engaging in some of these quirky or irritating behaviors or failing to take action in other positive ways that are addressed in this chapter are not in and of themselves sure signs that we may be "losing it." But I do believe that not being aware of some of this stuff can create a tendency on our parts to be a bit lazy, inattentive, and even careless about our societal and mental acuity—not a good thing when attempting to age gracefully, deliberately.

I am well aware that there are lots of reasons for our difficulties with decision making at times. Some decisions like when to sell our family homes, for example, are simply fundamentally difficult. But other factors play a role, as well: too much time on our hands after retirement, fear of change, unnecessary worrying, obsession with minutia, and many others. I am reminded of conversations with folks about cooking.

Some who really would like to become passionate about it but choose to stay away from it, they say, because they are afraid that they will make mistakes. Cooking is like just about everything else in life: mistakes should lead to learning and learning should lead to growth. I firmly believe that, if we pay attention and accept the fact that mistakes can and will happen, most fear about decision making can be overcome. The same can be said for taking chances by taking positive action when doing nothing seems safer. These are things that I have had to work through at times—occasionally with the help of a professional counselor.[40] The rewards for doing so, however, have been huge.

You may be able to make the changes that are necessary to make decisions and to take positive action on your own. Or, if you can only move on with the help of a counsellor, then get some help. In either case—when you are ready—move forward. You may also consider using as a mantra this little phrase that I first heard in the Navy: Lead, follow, or get out of the way...!

---

[40] I have had very little to say about the importance of seeking professional counseling when dealing with personal issues that may be overwhelming. This does not mean that I don't see counselling as important and valuable. I absolutely do. I know it works and I am a strong advocate for it.

**Impatience**

Yes, I know that I have already brought up the important topic/practice of patience a number of times already. I just thought I should simply mention it again here—for my sake—in light of my comments in this final chapter. Shall we move on?

**Imbalance**

Think Balance! 'Nuff said!!

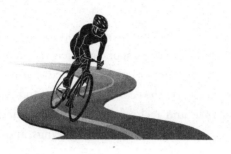

Chapter 10

# *Awareness: Keeping in Touch with Things that Matter*

I suppose that I could begin every chapter in this book by stating how important its subject is to aging deliberately. What I have to say in this chapter, however, *is* of particular importance. It is right up there with what we shared in Chapter 1 on attitude and outlook. Being aware is about growth and growing *up* with age, not *old* with it. In fact awareness is directly connected to attitude and outlook. To be aware is to be armed with knowledge, facts, truth. And to be aware is to push back against people or institutions who would make an effort to take advantage of our ignorance, to exploit us, to make us—dare I say it—*victims.* In the end, giving in to such things is giving up—the utter antithesis of aging deliberately.

Awareness is a huge subject, taking in just about everything we experience in life as we age. Consequently, to keep the topic manageable, I am going to approach it by discussing some of its most vital components (keeping in mind all of the time that they are all interrelated): current events (to include war and peace, the economy, the arts, and pop culture), politics, science and technology, our surroundings and the *moment,* the environment, other living beings, and our Selves, especially our health (physical, mental, and emotional). First, however, I need to say something about active versus passive awareness.

One could say that the simple act of noticing something and taking cognizance of it might pass for *awareness* of it and, thus, checking the awareness block; right? No … mere noticing and cognizance are not enough. Truly being aware, like just about everything else of importance, requires *effort.* And, by effort, I mean paying attention followed by thought and then some sort of response. This is especially important as we age. We need to push back against lethargy and complacency. We need to be ever mindful of replacing inertia with momentum. I have an example.

Virtually every weekday morning while having my coffee at about 7:30, I notice a particular car passing by my house at a speed which is obviously far in excess of the posted twenty-five mile per hour limit. (Speeding on my road is not, by the way, an unusual occurrence. The driver referred is just a repeat offender.) The speeding vehicle is easy to notice by residents and may even cause a reaction—say, anger—in most. Unfortunately, for many folks, however, the angry reaction, even though it is very likely to grow in intensity, is as far as it goes. In fact, the more often many of my neighbors—younger and older alike—notice the speeding car, the more they become angry about it. This relentless cycle of poor and dangerous driving on the part of the speeder followed by angry reactions on the parts of those who notice it, but who do nothing constructive or positive in *response,* is dangerous to the community. It is also disruptive to my neighbors' sense of wellbeing as safety concerns and unrelieved anger build up. Now, if I don't settle for passive awareness and, instead, turn what I have noticed into thoughtful and *active* awareness, I will be moved to respond. And, by responding (not reacting) with some form of positive action, I just may be able to *do* something about the problem—the speeding that is causing so much anxiety and anger. So ... what is to be done?

This is how I approached the issue. Over a week's time, I recorded the dates and times of the speeding along with a description of the car, including its license number (which took me several attempts to obtain because of the speed involved). During this period, I also prepared a petition that outlined the speeding problem in general and requested action of various types and obtained signatures from more than 75% of the adults who live on the same stretch of the road.[41] I followed up with a letter discussing both the repeat offender and the speeding problem in general along with the petition (sent snail mail). Some days later I paid a visit to the local police station and spoke with the police chief of this small community. In the letter and during my visit to the chief, I provided a calm, rational description of the issue and offered several reasonable solutions. I made a point of being objective and tactful but firm in my request for action. And action was, indeed taken: additional speed controls were installed and a significant number

---

[41] I should add here that most of the folks who signed the petition were delighted to participate but offered sincere skepticism that anything would be done by law enforcement in response.

of tickets were written over the following weeks. The speeding problem has not been completely resolved, but the situation is vastly improved.

I know what I just described sounds like what someone with too much time on his hands would do. But believe me; there are about a million things that I would rather spend my time on than this sort of thing. The point is that had I not taken this kind of action it is very likely that nothing would have been done about the problem—unless/until a someone (most likely a child) was hit on our road by a speeding driver. So, I think you can see how rather than stewing in anger and very likely eventually creating totally unnecessary emotional and possibly even physical health issues for yourself as a result, you can feel at ease and really good about helping to have resolved an issue confronting you and your neighbors by taking reasonable action, calmly pushing back, choosing *not* to be a victim.

I know that the previous example may seem a bit simplistic relative to the larger, much more dynamic subject of awareness. The fact of the matter, however, is that we all know lots of people who do notice things—many things—that are irritating and/or downright dangerous that certainly do create anxiety and anger for themselves and others. They become increasingly angry about the issue but choose to remain passive, unengaged. This inaction is neither helpful nor healthy; it *is* playing the role of victim. Being victimized by choice as we age is *not* aging deliberately. As you read what is to follow in the rest of this chapter, please keep the critical difference between passive and active awareness in mind and challenge yourself to consider how you can be more active in your awareness of all things in life.

**Awareness of Current Events**

Let's consider just a handful of the issues/events that are in the news or taking place as I write this subsection—some or all of which I sincerely hope are resolved to some degree by the time this book is published. Locally and at the state level, infrastructure (specifically, the condition of our roads and fresh water supply, especially in Flint, Michigan) is a really big deal. But many of us are also concerned about the plight of the six hundred and fifty or so gray wolves in the upper peninsula of the state who may be subjected to a new state law that would allow hunters to have at them. Regionally, the looming possibility that the incredibly invasive Asian carp could invade the Great Lakes, fracking, and the fate of the once booming and now crumbling city of Detroit come to mind. Nationally, the economy is always a matter of great significance, as is drought in the west and some plains states, as is gun violence, as is the racial divide that remains such a huge and deeply divisive issue—whether we choose to admit it or get serious about dealing with it or not. Globally, Ebola, Zika, and other horrible epidemics (and the ignorance of so many with respect to them), climate change, terrorist groups like the "Islamic State" and the carnage they leave in their wake, and the greed, lack of opportunity, and intolerance that cripples so many societies—and especially the women within them—are almost mind-numbing in their importance and complexity.

On a lighter note, I have become convinced that it is also important to be aware of what is going on in the world of pop culture. Whether the subject is music, television shows, movies, graphic art, dress, hair styles, language, or just about anything else that is trendy, knowing what is happening matters. And I think the main reason that it matters is the effort that it takes to be and to stay in touch with the things and people that are having an effect on the thinking, attention, buying habits, and loves of all folks—both old *and* young. Doing so keeps us engaged, caring—one way or the other—about the world, keeps us thinking, keeps us active, keeps us *alive*. I am certainly not saying we need to try to *like* everything that is new and trendy. God knows I don't. But I do think we need to know enough about what is happening in pop culture to have an educated, thoughtful opinion about something's artistic or cultural merit. Staying engaged in this regard is also a very good way to prevent ourselves from getting wrapped up in what I have already referred to as "generational warfare." When we notice something, anything in life that we don't understand, it can frighten us. When things frighten or confuse us (often because of our ignorance), we often react negatively. A good although perhaps tired example is the way many in my generation originally reacted (and continue to react) to RAP music. I have heard folks around my age say on scores of occasions things like "I like just about any music … just as long as it isn't *RAP*." When I have asked them why, their answers are often alarmingly over simplified and harsh: "It's a bunch of crap"; or "It makes no sense"; or "I can't understand it"; or "It's all about sex, drugs, and violence." Not only are such responses inaccurate; they are also unfair. If sixty-somethings would simply take the time and make the effort to really listen to artists like Common or Eminem or Nick Cannon, I think they may start to see how poetic, insightful, and generally relevant some RAP music can be. Again, the point is not to try to get everyone within ten or fifteen years of my age to love RAP music or the larger hip-hop subculture; the real key is taking the time and making the effort to give things a chance and to base opinions on real experience with and thought about something rather than making ignorant, biased, reactionary condemnations because something is different.

Does it really matter if you and I have taken the time to gain at least some familiarity with the most significant people and issues of our day? And when I say "some familiarity…" I am talking about knowing something more than what a certain favorite TV or radio pundit may have to say about something. I mean taking the time to get the facts, the truth and then to give the matter some considered thought. Of course it matters. It is the responsibility of each of us to be aware/informed of the issues of the day. And it also is good for our minds to learn about what is happening, give it some considered thought, and develop positions on those matters which will, in turn, affect how we act socially and … politically.

**Awareness of Politics**

Regardless of your feelings about politics and/or politicians, maintaining an active awareness of what is going on politically on the local, regional, national, and global stages is more than staying informed; it is a key component to being a responsible, contributing, ethical member of society—no matter how frustrated you may become or how satisfied you may be with the status quo. As I write this subsection on Election Day, 2014, I have several important election-related questions at the back of my mind: Will the Republican Party take control of the US Senate and, if they do, what will (or won't) happen as a result? Who will win the very tight Governor's race in my home state of Michigan? How will what happens today affect the 2106 Presidential election? How many people who vote today have any idea of what the issues really are or truly understand the proposals and initiatives they will find on their ballots? And how many folks simply won't vote at all for any number of reasons ranging from apathy to lack of the appropriate ID card?

I am not one of those who believe that voting for every office up for grabs or every proposal on the ballot is necessarily an obligation on every single Election Day or something that is required to be a good citizen. Frankly, I would rather see folks make the thoroughly considered decision *not* to vote on any given office or issue if they think that an occasional abstention on a given race or proposal is consistent with a political point they wish to make. Simply completing a ballot without having a clue what one is doing simply to say they voted or blindly following some voting tradition that they have followed for years is obviously not within the definition of political activism. The point is to be *aware* of the political local, regional, national, and global landscapes with all of their complications, nuances, and potential. Being aware takes time and effort and thought and action and occasionally, yes, considered *inaction*. For our purposes, the role of political awareness vis-à-vis aging deliberately is staying *involved*, allowing for possibility, and not letting cynicism, inertia, or downright mental or physical laziness stand in the way of thoughtful respect for others' *reasoned* beliefs and opinions.[42] It also involves action—whether at the voting booth or possibly in the streets when an active, nonviolent, political response is a way to help institute meaningful political change.[43]

---

[42] I no more feel obliged to respect ill-conceived, hateful, ignorant political opinion than I do respecting "elders" simply because they are older. For example, I do not respect Senator James Inhofe's position that climate change is a "hoax." And I do not respect old fuddy duddies who are consistently nasty and rude because their "old age" entitles them to be.

[43] Is it better to obey an ethically corrupt law (those associated with segregation,

Notwithstanding the virtues inherent in the occasional protest non-vote, I also believe in the lesser-of-two-evils voting strategy: If the only two (or more) choices are less than great, choosing the least bad one on election day does make a certain amount of sense to me. The point, once again, is to make the effort to be informed/aware enough to make intelligent, well-considered political decisions ... and then, in most cases, to take the time to vote. As you can see, political awareness is much more than being engaged on one day every couple of years to vote. Doing so is like calling oneself a Christian and going to church twice a year—on Easter and Christmas Eve. Political awareness is political activism and the activism is what keeps folks—aging folks—tuned in, alert, relevant, and deliberate. While I probably will not go out and sit in at the state capital building tomorrow if my folks aren't elected and/or the proposals I support are not passed, I am neither too cynical nor too old to take it to the streets if the need arises—not to prove that I am still able to do so, but rather to take meaningful political action based upon reasoned and *active* awareness.[44]

## Awareness of science and technology

Not to put too fine an edge on it ... I am quite good with science but I am still attempting to get myself into the Twenty First Century with regard to technology. Once again, I would

---

for example) or to break the law and so foster positive political change? I think the answer to that one is clear.

[44] I am reminded of the case, which I just heard about today, of an eighty-one year old man from Oklahoma who was running for Congress as a Democrat in an overwhelmingly Republican district. He never made it to Election Day; he died the day before from injuries that he sustained in an automobile accident previously. The irony of all this was certainly not lost on me; nor was the beauty of his willingness to be politically positive, active, and ... *deliberate* up to the end.

argue that it *is* important—*very* important—to stay in touch
with the latest … stuff. I pretty much missed the techno-boat
about thirty years ago and have been struggling to catch up
ever since. My problem back in the eighties was that I just
never cared to get the basics. And as things started to move
ahead—pretty much without me—I fell further and further
behind as technological developments and advances moved
forward at faster and faster speed. These days I am narrowing
the gap … and I am happy about that just because it is keeping
me in the game—mentally. But the fact of the matter is that
if we want to be efficient and if we wish to … matter, we need
to communicate as well as we possibly can. Understanding the
technology of communication is a must. Awareness of all that
is at our disposal to reach out to others—quickly and effectively—is central, I believe, to aging deliberately.

### Awareness of our surroundings and of the moment

Although I am not going to devote pages to this, I do want
to emphasize the huge importance of being aware of our surroundings. This means putting down the cell phones and pulling the buds out of our ears and doing our best to use all of our
senses as much as we possibly can. My best brief anecdote to
express how I feel about using all of our senses is this: Teaching
my classes in person, not on line. While I am no enemy of
technology and fully understand the importance and beauty of
distance learning—especially for working parents—I say, with
all respect to my distance-learning teaching colleagues, it is not
for me. The reason, as I put it, is that I need to activate *all* of my
senses when I teach: sight, hearing, touching, even smelling.
As I tell folks, I know I can see and hear my students on line,
but I need to *smell* them. I am not trying to be perverse here;

I am trying to underscore the importance of using all of our senses to be as aware of and in touch with our surroundings as possible. This is something that has become more and more important to me as I have aged—deliberately.

## Awareness of the environment

We could also call this subsection "Awareness of the Future." I know that we could—for hours and hours—debate the most important issue regarding our future and, so, our present. No matter what someone who pays attention to things might choose as the top three, I'll bet the environment will be somewhere in there. So, if we cannot agree that the environment is *the* most important issue, let's agree that it is enormously important.

Just what does "awareness of the environment" mean and how does it relate to aging deliberately? I am going to address the first part of the question directly and hope that my answer to that will, in large part, deal with the second part. Being aware of the environment means being aware of *everything*. No, I am not attempting to be glib; I really mean it. Every time we start our car to drive down the street to the store—instead of walking or riding our bikes—we have done something that affects the environment. Each time we use paper or plastic[45] rather than a re-useable canvas bag to pack up our groceries

---

[45] I just have to add something here—about plastic bags. First of all, it is not just about their appearance just about everywhere they should not be—including in the stomachs of sea turtles and around the necks of birds. They are also made with petroleum—lots and lots of it ... an estimated twelve million barrels of oil each year. If I had any hair, I would pull clumps of it out every time I see people (often young ones with children who should really be concerned about such things) asking for double plastic bags in which to place their gallon-sized jugs of milk. You know; the ones that already have a handle. Give us a break, folks!

we have done something that affects the environment. The same goes for playing golf rather than going for a walk, using a garbage disposal rather than composting, drying our clothes in a dryer rather than on a clothesline, letting the water run constantly while we are brushing our teeth, mindlessly killing a snake or a spider or a bat just because they are what they are, or thousands of other things, we are affecting our environment … negatively. Conversely, just about every time we plant a tree, turn down or, better, turn *off* our air conditioners, install solar grids, save a bat from being caught in someone's home, do good things for honey bees, clean up some polluted pond, stream, or lake, and countless other constructive acts, we are affecting the environment … positively. The point is that each of us really *can* do things that either negatively or positively affect the environment, and it is our awareness of this followed by our choice to do something in response that matters—no matter what anyone else does or does not do. I think you can see that deliberateness comes into play in environmental awareness and how actually *doing* small, consistent positive things as a result of that awareness as we age helps give meaning to our lives and just may serve as a really good example for younger folks to follow.

### Awareness of other living things

Obviously, this one is closely tied to the previous one, and I am going way beyond awareness of friends and family members here. I am talking about being aware of *all* living things: human and non-human beings, flowers, tress, the works …. And, by "awareness," I am, once again, thinking of consideration, reflection, and respect. I am talking about actually stopping to think about cutting down that old tree in the front yard that tends to create "too much shade" for the grass and/or drops "too many leaves" in the fall. Perhaps the life of the tree could be spared by planting (or not planting) something else that does not require light under the tree and by using all of its wonderful fallen leaves as compost rather than grudgingly blowing them into a pile and setting them on fire—with all the resultant smoke and nasty release of $CO_2$.

I have already made my point about creepy, crawly, and/or flying things that can sting or bite (e.g., snakes, spiders, bats, wasps, and bees): We need to leave them alone—just because we should. Never mind the fact that most of these non-human animals are really good for all of us—by pollinating, keeping other invasive things in check, and hundreds of other generally cool, environmentally friendly things. And let's not forget about the treatment of non-human things while they are with us: many zoo and circus animals, chickens at poultry and egg production factories, and especially Asian elephants who are tortured into submissive behavior in order for folks to get a ride and their keepers a buck or two. And being kind, generous, and considerate in our relations with *human* animals is something that may need a bit more of our attention than we normally give it, as well. Once again, I am not trying to advocate for sainthood for us; I am arguing for thought, reflection, and considered responses (rather than reactions) when inter-reacting with all other living things—even if it means taking out a mosquito, or a cockroach, or some other creature whose very existence may be an issue for us or some other human or non-human animal.

## Awareness of our Selves

I could have started with this but chose to leave it for the end. You see, everything about aging deliberately begins and ends with our Selves. It is ultimately all about being aware of each and every thing that we do—not to the extent of obsessively focusing on our every thought and action, but in a general sense and in advance. If we make a practice of being in touch with our Selves, we know that paying attention to our relationships with others, our breathing, our sleeping, our weight, our senses, our ability to find humor in almost everything, our appreciation of beauty, our mental processes, the things that we eat and drink, our kindness and consideration, and the healthiness of our minds and our bodies is not only important but actually the essence of *Being*. And this awareness—beginning and ending with Self—will also make our interrelationships with just about everyone and everything measurably more meaningful and fulfilling. Here is an arguably simple (I am hopeful not simplistic) example. Let's say you decide to go for a nice walk. It is a beautiful fall day and there is a wonderful wooded path that passes along a lovely rushing stream nearby. So ... off you go. Here's the deal: Are you ready to enjoy the entirety of the walk or are you allowing the beauty of the moment to be bombarded by thoughts of the boss you are not particularly fond of or your perceived need of a new, flashier car that may need some creative financing to own? Do you pack your iPod and plug in as you take your first couple of steps and, in doing so, focus some of your most important sensors on something other than each wonder-filled component of the walk? Or, do you do your Self a favor and revitalize all that is in you by taking in the sights, the sounds, the smells, the textures of everything that you can allow in? Do you choose to hear your breathing, your footsteps, the sounds of the water, the chattering of the squirrels, the wind whispering through the remaining colorful leaves in the trees, the calls of the birds, perhaps even the last buzzing of the bees that still may have a few things to tend to before the onset of the cold weather? Are you aware of the caterpillars that are hurrying across the path to avoid your feet and other living things that may want them for lunch? Can you sense the autumn sun breaking through the treetops and giving your exposed skin a little added warmth? Are you *aware* that being *aware* of all of these things is actually being *aware* of those wonderful senses of your Self that tune you into Life *itself*? This, I think, is the essence of becoming comfortable—really comfortable—in our own skins and getting the most out of, well … everything, as we learn and grow and age.

And while we are at it—this important business of being aware of our Selves—let's not forget about taking really good care of the most important home that each of us has: our bodies. I have already alluded to this and will do so more later. I just want to end this chapter on Awareness with a reminder about body maintenance. Some of us may not have had such a reminder since we heard it from our parents. I'm talking about making sure that our skin stays healthy, our teeth are brushed and flossed, our sight and hearing are not neglected, our bodies stay hydrated, that we get enough sleep and exercise, and that we keep our love lives healthy and vibrant. I know that you know that each of these is as vital as anything else is in our quest to age deliberately. Sometimes a little prodding does a world of good. Let's consider ourselves prodded.

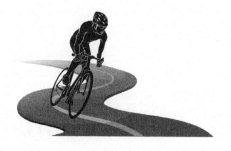

Chapter 11

# Work and Volunteering: Remaining Productive

For me, other than health and family,[46] there is nothing more important in life than work and its close cousin—volunteering. I have not forgotten faith or my spiritual side which I know are at the top of the lists of many folks. I acknowledge and celebrate this, but they are simply not in my top three. Note, too, I use the term "work" and not "job." Those of us who are lucky enough to have a job should be grateful, but a job is often simply a way to earn a living. A job can be annoying, boring, regimented, spirit numbing, downright disgusting, any or all of the above, and ... even worse. How many times have you heard someone say something like this: "Man, I hate my job!"? One's *work*, however, now that is an altogether different thing from a job. Have you *ever* heard

---

[46] And here I include significant others and extremely close friends as "family." More on this in Chapter 14.

someone say "Man, I hate my *work!*"? I am guessing not. Our work can give us sustenance, meaning, fulfillment, intellectual and/or physical challenges and it can exhaust us. And, if we are fortunate enough to truly love our jobs and can look at them as our life's work, well that is just about as good as it can get.

Occasionally, I like to reflect on all the jobs I have had in my life—any activity for which I was paid that was something other than a one-shot deal—and think about which ones were really fun and which ones were a real drag. I have been a janitor, a child sitter, a lawn guy, a sporting goods store worker, a security guard at a girl's dorm and a resident advisor during my undergraduate days, a regular member of a product-testing panel, a library staff member, a dairy worker (cottage cheese, sour cream, ice cream, etc.), a truck driver, a furniture mover, a graduate teaching assistant, a high-school substitute teacher, a law clerk, an editor, a writer, a lawyer and naval officer, a college/university-level instructor and administrator, and I probably held several other jobs that I no longer remember. It is interesting to note that the job I most disliked was very closely tied to the job (my life's work) that I loved most. I detested substitute teaching (mainly because I felt that I was so utterly ineffective at walking into a high school classroom and actually getting some real teaching done) and I loved and love to this day teaching my own classes of college/university level composition, literature, law, and humanities. The real work in my life includes my career in the US Navy (twenty-four years) and academics and, more recently, editing and writing. While I was an attorney during my entire navy career, it was the service and leadership component of my job that kept me going and fulfilled—much more than the lawyering component. As for academics and, more specifically, teaching … let's just say it is in my DNA; it is what I am about. And as for editing and writing, we shall see.

Now, this brings up an interesting issue. Using my definition of a job which contemplates both some level of routine and some level of compensation, I would like to consider and compare an occupation—really hard, challenging *work*, perhaps the most difficult thing to do really well—that can be more rewarding than just about anything imaginable and pays nothing monetarily: *Parenting*. While I have never been a father, I have had tastes of parenting as a mentor and/or surrogate to several young folks. But, as much as these relationships have meant and still mean to me, they just aren't the same as being an adoptive[47] or natural parent. Nevertheless, parenting is work that I have observed carefully for many years and fundamentally respect and admire when it is done well—not necessarily perfectly but patiently and ... deliberately. I have watched with awe as really wonderful patience, caring, teaching, and love are poured into children consistently over years and I have also been horrified at what I have seen as indifferent, continually angry, impatient keepers of children consistently neglect, abandon, and abuse this most important work and the children on the other end of it. For my money, nothing rivals the difficulty or the rewards of excellent 24/7 parenting; and it doesn't stop once the children reach a certain age. I will have more to say about parenting and family and their relationships to each other and to aging deliberately in Chapter 14. But now I would like to turn to another type of work or job (the term chosen for it will likely depend on how one feels about its value, worth, and fulfillment): homemaking or being a house husband/house wife, if you like.

---

[47] I would include long-term legal guardianships here as well.

Since, for the moment, I am currently a family of one, my homemaking is not particularly demanding. While I really do enjoy it, I regard it as a non-paying *job*—mainly because there are other things that involve my labor that I am more dedicated to. For me, homemaking is more of an avocation than a vocation. There are, however, lots of folks—with or without children—for whom homemaking is pretty much a full time occupation. And, given a chance to differentiate between job and work as we are using the terms here, homemakers would probably be consistent only in their inconsistency of how they view such labor. In any case, folks who *do* regard homemaking as their life's work are likely to do it well and take a great deal of pride in it.

My point in the discussion of work so far is to celebrate whatever it is that we do when we are not sleeping, eating, recreating, or involved in things that are not our work. And by celebrating what it is that we do and what others do, we recognize the extraordinary importance of work in our lives. The more cognizant we are of the significance of work, the more we are rewarded by it—whether we are nineteen or ninety. And if we are fortunate to stay working until we *choose* no longer to do so, we are truly lucky, indeed. While I am not working (i.e., teaching) at the present time, I have every intention of getting back to it in the not too distant future. Frankly, I can't wait to get back into the classroom and, once I have found a place and a position that is right for me, I can't imagine walking away from it. Work in the form of teaching is a necessity for me. It keeps me engaged, in touch, thinking, and growing. In other words, work helps me to be a deliberate ager.

Since 9/11, the military has become the subject of much admiration in the United States; Americans are unabashedly thankful for what service members do. First responders—especially firefighters and emergency medical personnel—are also very highly regarded.[48] Even if some folks have issues with certain doctors, lots of lawyers, and some other professionals, most Americans will at least give them credit for most of what they do—if not their normally much higher than average pay checks. Teachers get the respect but not the financial support that most of us think they deserve, and then there are the professional athletes and successful musicians and actors whose salaries seem always to be a source of eye rolling but whose status is usually greatly admired. As for politicians, especially members of Congress, I am not one to condemn all of them—not by a long shot. But the fourteen percent approval rating Congress is currently receiving makes the view of the average American about what they do and how they do it pretty clear ... not good. Yet there are so many of us who do *not* necessarily have high profile or hugely admired work but who simply go about doing what we do in a competent and occasionally inspired manner each day of the work week and sometimes beyond that into our off-duty time. In fact, I think we have all read stories about or have actually known people who have seemingly mundane unappealing jobs who turn those jobs into their life's work by throwing all that they can into being the best janitor, crossing guard, cashier, house cleaner, or store greeter that they can be. Sometimes I think that I especially admire and respect these folks with the least desirable jobs for doing their work really well and with great pride each and every day.

---

[48] Police officers—despite the bad press some have been given recently (justifiably or not) also enjoy respect, gratitude, and appreciation for what they do from most folks.

Someone who really grasped the importance of work was one of my favorite people of the last hundred years: Studs Terkel. And, by far, one of my favorite works of nonfiction was his book, *Working*, published in 1975. The book's subtitle provides a not-so-subtle clue about the specific subject matter of this wonderful piece of *work*: People talk about what they do all day and how they feel about what they do. Studs interviewed scores of folks—everyone from cops to prostitutes and professionals to hard laborers—who open up about their work and what it means to them. The most important thing that I took away from reading the book was the huge significance work plays in so many of our lives—even for those folks who were not particularly enthralled with what they were doing for work at the time they were interviewed. It also has made me think what it must mean to so many people—all over the world—who simply have no work. How lost and empty they must feel not to be able to contribute, to create something someone else will buy, to have a calling that can actually put a roof over their heads and food on their tables, to be part of … the *working* world. Should it be surprising to us when we see young men (in particular) joining gangs or terrorist groups if, for no other reason, simply to have some cause to be a part of, to have something to *do* that might even *pay* them for their efforts? This, by no means, is any sort of acceptance of the evil that is created by those who have given up trying other ways to earn a living and to gain respect. I mention this as simply another way of illustrating just how fundamentally important work is to so many of us humans.

I think that—for most folks who *can*—work is as important to the human experience as almost anything. Those of us who have work—especially work that we truly love—know commitment, dedication, pride, fulfillment, independence, and at least some self-sufficiency. No matter how sustaining and rewarding our work can be, it is not going to help us age deliberately, however, if it is out of balance with the other important components of our lives: family and friends, spirituality, health. I am sure that all of us know or have read about folks whose work is *everything* to them.[49] They eat, drink, sleep, and *live* their work. Family, health, and spirituality barely have a place in their lives. The drive of these folks may come from ego, obsession, financial gain, fear of failure, and/or any number of other things. They may think their total dedication to their work is what makes them happy and, to a certain extent, they may be correct. But what a way to live—so utterly out of balance. These are folks who have choices in life and, like others who choose to let things get terribly out of balance in their lives, life itself becomes one-dimensional. These are folks who do not *grow* as they age; they often simply become old and then they die … long after their humanity and their joy predeceased their physical deaths. I know this all may sound judgmental; it is not meant to be. I just want to be clear on the point that, no matter how important work is to life, it is deadly to our essence if it *becomes* life. So, here is to good hard work balanced with all of the other key components of a full rich life: love, health, family and friends, and the spiritual.

For those of us who do have a choice and can find other things than work to do with the time we are not sharing with our friends and families and/or recreating and/or staying

---

[49] I'm not referring to folks who *must* work from sunup to sundown virtually every day just to feed, house, and clothe their families (the subsistence farmer in the Philippines, for example). For these folks, family and spirituality are enormously important parts of their lives; they simply have little choice in what they can do each day *other* than to work to live.

fit, volunteering (and here I am talking about spending time with causes that benefit others—human and non-human animals, trees, parks, waterways, etc.—and for which there is no compensation) may be yet another enriching, fulfilling, and worthwhile activity that can add a wonderful dimension to life. The beauty of volunteering is that it can take just about any form we choose. I have gladly taken on volunteering projects ranging from coaching Babe Ruth baseball and women's softball to teaching college English courses (gratis) at the college where I used to work as an administrator to working with the Jackson, Michigan, local Personal Care Ministry which distributes personal necessity items to those in need. And I have been fortunate to work with a number of other volunteer organizations over the last few decades as well.

Those who have been involved with volunteering often find it as rewarding as what they do or retired from doing for their life's work. It is engaging and usually very productive; it is *always* appreciated. And another benefit of volunteering is that it keeps us involved, active, in touch, and aware. I'm sure I don't need to do any (additional) salesmanship on behalf of this enriching pastime; I just felt that I could not ignore it when discussing some of the really positive things that help us to age deliberately. The win-win associated with volunteering should be obvious as should be the need. No matter what we do in life that involves work (and volunteering), if we love it and dedicate a significant but sustainable (i.e., balanced) portion of our lives to it, it will love us back and will help us to grow and age … deliberately.

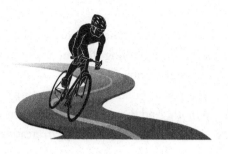

Chapter 12

# Hobbies and Other Fun Stuff

This is supposed to be a light, fun chapter, so let's not get too wrapped up in definitions here. I suppose the word hobby can mean lots of things to lots of people. Generally speaking, a hobby is something we do for fun on a fairly regular basis—usually (perhaps best) done in our leisure time. You know … after the wood has been corded, the fields plowed, the cows milked, and the children cared for. I like to think of hobbies this way. If life is a meal, hobbies are the desert—certainly not required but ahhhh soooo good! In any case, hobbies are for us and our fellow travelers, a time for recreation—a time to re-create ourselves through fun and relaxation.

My point here is that whether we are completely retired, working part-time, or still at it forty-plus hours a week, there should be some time each week for us to do something other than life's necessities—even if we truly love our work and other parts of the "main course" of our lives. I should note here that I consider volunteering (discussed in the previous chapter as well) to be a very good candidate for a hobby but only if you really enjoy it as something that you really want to do. It doesn't count if you feel obligated.

Hobbies can test us in many ways—exercising our bodies, our minds,[50] or both. And that's a good thing. Many of us thrive on challenge even during our hobby time/recreation time. The key to challenging hobbies is to embrace the challenge and eschew the stress that can accompany it if we let it. Traveling comes to mind as a hobby (one of mine) that can test us mentally or physically or even both simultaneously. In the last few years, I have taken three long trips[51] of varying lengths (ten months, thirteen months, and ten weeks), and I am here to tell you that long multi-country journeys can be hard work, challenging, taxing, and, yes, even stressful at times. But, heck, even more every-day activities like cycling can be stressful at times as we dodge inattentive drivers, having to lay our bicycles down occasionally to evade vehicular contact. Despite the occasional stress, hobbies that may push us a bit are just fine with me.

The point is to be engaged, to get away from the norm in whatever way suits us because doing so keeps us sharp and, in one way or another, in shape. And how healthy hobbies differ! For example, I have friends who participate in Renaissance Fairs—yes, all the costumes and affectations. They love it because they really get into it—constantly doing research,

---

[50] I know that many of you have hobbies that are both fun and really good for the brain. Reading is probably the most obvious. But there are many others that come to mind: crossword puzzles, Sudoku, Scrabble, Words with Friends are just a few. I find that writing pushes me mentally and helps me to keep my edge. I have also started playing mind exercise games such as Luminosity and Sheppard Software Brain Games, and I recommend these and any other activity that keeps you thinking and engaged—especially important as we add years.

[51] One of them (the second) is at the heart of the first of my "deliberately" books: *Traveling Deliberately.*

planning their next venue, sharing stories with friends. This is definitely not for me. But I get it; it provides a balance for them and so it works.

Let me remove whatever mystery may be out there regarding what my hobbies are. As you now know, travel is an important hobby of mine although I think my long-term, multi-country journeying may be slowing down—if only because Barbara is now so much more part of my life and she prefers less involved travel. And this is all good with me. That said, a trip to Tanzania to try a Mt. Kilimanjaro climb remains in the works. But we are talking about a relatively brief couple of weeks in Africa.

I also consider writing to be much more a hobby (an avocation) than a job. Teaching (especially English composition, American literature, and health law) is another one which, the way I do it, is both mentally and physically taxing. I also consider many forms of physical exercise to be hobbies. No more running or tennis … or golf! Now it's cycling, kayaking, canoeing, work outs, yard work, and WALKING (perhaps my favorite) among others. I also love to cook, am interested and involved in politics, and consider myself an amateur geographer and historian. I really enjoy (classical) music, art, the theater, and movies but so do most people. Since I am not a musician or a painter or a sculptor or an actor, I'm not sure my mere enjoyment of these things makes them "hobbies" of mine. (But, then again, we are not quibbling over definitions in this chapter.) Strangely enough considering my academic background, I am not an omnivorous reader and take on maybe two or three novels a year. This is simply a matter of my priorities and time, not any kind of a statement about the relative importance of reading.

So… what does all of this have to do with aging deliberately? I have been planting clues all along: attitude, engagement, mental and physical health, fun, BALANCE …. And much of this goes back to what I had to say in Chapter 1 about attitude and outlook. I am talking about staying fresh, having and being fun, taking it all in without being manic about stuff. Hobbies are a component of the whole of aging deliberately. They reward us for our hard work—at the job, as parents, as contributors. And I think they have the potential for not only helping to keep us mentally, emotionally, and physically fit at our respective ages, but they can also contribute to a quality, happy, positive, and even longer life. I am not certain about the science behind it all, but I have seen healthy hobbies/recreation do wonders for me and plenty of other folks.

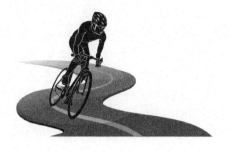

Chapter 13

# Finances: Keeping Cash Flow Realistic and Low on Stress

This chapter is not about how to make and keep millions of dollars. I am no expert on such things and have no desire to be. I just have a few things to say about keeping the fiscal house in order without requiring masses of cash to do so. As a matter of fact, I really do believe that being preoccupied with finances and maintenance of lots of stuff is not healthy and certainly no way for most of us to age deliberately. Simply too much stress in it.

So, let me offer three interconnecting key notions with a brief discussion of each to be the focus of this chapter: planning; budget; and, of course, balance.

**Planning**
It's never too late. I have two sets of married-couple friends who worked hard for years and had some good luck and,

consequently, established an excellent income and an impressive array of assets. Unfortunately, a run of losses, some overreaching (aka speculation), and unexpected expenses have left them scrambling. Family dynamics—more than a few players, each with their own intelligence and will—have played and continue to play an important role in the difficulties. Whatever financial plan had been in place for these couples has been overcome by events. What I see happening now is lots of reacting—lots of half-baked strategies but no effective big-picture plan. I am also detecting in these fifty-something and sixty-something friends a sense of despair, a feeling that the good days are past and all that can be hoped for now is an "existence." I understand the disappointment but I do not embrace the settling. Sure, the days of bigger than, faster than, more of everything may be over, but as I have learned by intentionally down-sizing and simplifying—out of choice, not necessity—cutting the unnecessary extras out and embracing the essentials is, in a word, liberating. Embracing a lifestyle that is understood, appreciated, and under control is, I truly believe, an essential ingredient in lowering stress, staying active, loving life, and, ultimately, aging deliberately.

This is yet another place where what I have to say in Chapter 1 ("Attitude"), Chapter 4 ("Eating and Drinking"), and Chapter 5 ("Fitness") comes into play. The point is, that if a change in lifestyle and/or plans is a financial necessity or a financially unnecessary desire, your outlook and your physical and psychological/emotional condition will serve you greatly in refocusing and having the energy and vision to develop a new plan—one that incorporates the truly important things in life like emotional and physical well-being, low stress, and the nurturing of loving relationships. Being willing to make and then to act on a new financial plan is necessary because so many of us find ourselves in our forties, fifties, sixties, and beyond in so vast an array of circumstances—many of which are far different than we may have imagined only a few years earlier. That said, a focus on simplifying and shedding the so-called trappings of "success" allows us to clear the air and develop a plan for the future that we can live with.[52]

Your plan first requires a (re)prioritization of your values and goals. After giving this serious consideration during a time when stress, emotional dynamics, and fiscal considerations are as stable as they can be, you will be ready to create it. Your revised plan may be very different or just a slightly tweaked version of the one currently in effect. The key is the thinking and soul-searching involved in the process. By the way, as much as I trust my own thinking and feelings, I count on the advice of a few people (not necessarily close friends and/or family members) whose opinions I trust and value and seek it out when making many of my financial and other important decisions. Sometimes I am simply too close to something of major significance to see it clearly, and sharing my vision and plans with trusted others is extraordinarily helpful. Once the new plan has been established and in place, I immediately begin the process of making notes on how I may keep the plan consistent with my vision—as life changes, variables come into

---

[52] This is certainly familiar territory for me. In my early fifties, I had an excellent income as a successful Navy attorney and adjunct college instructor. At one point, I owned two large, expensive boats, a home, and a Mercedes. Over the course of a few years, retirement from the Navy, and a change in location, I began to sense the folly inherent in the acquisition of things. In a matter of weeks, I decided to change plans, liquidate, and travel. This was doubtless one of the very best decisions I have ever made. I still find myself smiling to myself about it!

play, and dynamics make their impact on my plan, my values, my loved ones, and me.

All of this planning is a grand thing in aligning financial wants and needs with income, but without actually setting these things down in a real-world budget that can be consistently maintained without becoming enslaved by it we end up back where we started. So let's have a look at how one person's important but not terribly complicated life-style changes were turned into a new budget (AFTER) that was similar in design to the old one (BEFORE) but quite different in scope and emphasis. I will offer an example whose numbers closely reflect my own financial situation, even if my family situation is a little different.

### Budget[53]

As I suggested earlier, the planning is the fun part. Developing a reasonable budget to fit the plan is the difficult part. Budgeting is difficult because it takes research, careful consideration, soul-searching, and willingness to stay reasonably within it once it has been established. Developing a budget is also as much art as it is science because an effective, practical budget has factored within it what could happen as well as what is happening at the time it is developed.

Consider an upper middle class couple—each of whom contribute to family income of $10,300/month, net. (No children and/or no routine children-rearing expenses are in the mix.)

---

[53] I know that it will come as no surprise to many of you that some folks—folks with families, no less—run their finances with virtually no real plan, let alone an actual budget. Every day, week, month, and year ends—by hook or crook—with no major debt, lots of financial issues ... and stress, or an embarrassment of riches that could be put to better use. Perhaps you are one of these folks. If you are, it's time for a C change!

BEFORE:

Three thousand sq. ft. house in relatively upscale neighborhood

House value $400,000 (80K + 20K—Down Payment + Equity)

| | |
|---|---|
| Monthly Mortgage (P&I) | $2200 |
| Insurance | 150 |
| Taxes | 350 |
| Essential Maintenance/Repairs | 300 |
| Utilities | 300 |
| Food | 800 |
| Cars:      Mercedes Sedan Payment | 350 |
|            Jeep SUV Payment | 250 |
| Ins. | 280 |
| Gas | 220 |
| Maintenance | 100 |
| Club Membership(s) & Spending | 500 |
| Pool Maintenance | 150 |
| Ins.- Health, Dental, Life | 400 |
| Misc. Household Expenses | 600 |
| Yard Maintenance | 125 |
| Boat      (Payment) | 350 |
|           (Maintenance) | 150[54] |
|           (Slip) | 400 |
|           (Ins.) | 100 |
| Misc. Spending | 2100 |
| Travel | 0 |
| Long-Term Savings | 125 |
| *Total Spending* | *$10300* |

---

[54]  Of course, one blown engine can (and did) throw the boat owner over(board) budget.

AFTER:

| | |
|---|---|
| Rental apartment/house | $2000 |
| Utilities | 150 |
| Food | 800 |
| Car (used Toyota Corolla purchased for cash) | 0 |
| Car Insurance | 90 |
| Gas | 135 |
| Public Transportation | 150 |
| Other Insurance | 300 |
| Misc. Household Expenses | 300 |
| Yard | 0 |
| Pool—Apartment complex has a pool | 0 |
| Boat—no boat (other than kayak/canoe) | 0 |
| Misc. Spending | 2200 |
| Travel | 2100 |
| Long-Term Savings | 2075 |
| *Total Spending* | *$10300* |

**Balance**

Note that the BEFORE budget has so much more stuff—stuff to maintain more important stuff, stuff to continue to pay for, stuff to distract me from other really fun things like travel, exercise, and even sleep. The good news is that my BEFORE budget was, at least, a budget—that I was good about maintaining. The bad news was that its allowances for all of that unnecessary stuff and complications in my life left almost no time or money for travel and almost no monthly contributions to long-term savings. To be sure, the AFTER budget—representative of my current situation—is a far cry from what Henry David Thoreau was about at Walden (living deliberately in a simple cabin that he built at a pond in the woods for two years two months and two days in the 1850s). The concept of a simplification process, however, is crucial here—not necessarily the degree of it. Just to further illustrate my point about stuff accumulation a wee bit more, I offer you this glimpse of Americana which first struck me when I was living in Sunnyvale, California, in 1984. It seemed that my wife and I were the only folks who parked their cars in the garage. House after house in our neighborhood was displaying at least one but more often two or even three vehicles in their driveways or on the curbside in front of the residence. It didn't take us long to figure it out: stuff. Garage after garage was filled with stuff. I vowed there and then never to get to the point of displacing a vehicle from its proper place in the garage for the sake of acquisition and storage of stuff. I had to learn my lesson about acquisition of expensive cars and boats, large houses, and club memberships later. But I did learn; I simplified; and I love the change! Please give stuff-shedding and life style simplification some serious consideration. Budgeting and finances will certainly become far less challenging, and aging deliberately—without the constant stress and hassles of maintaining unnecessary stuff—will be far less difficult to establish and sustain.

At the outset of this chapter, I told you that, for me, dealing with finances while aging deliberately comes down to three essentials—planning; budget; and balance. I have spent a few pages dealing specifically with the planning and budgeting components. It seems to me the key ingredient of balance is implicit in both the essence and actual discussion of what I have had to say. Now, your sense of balance is, of course, not going to lead you to the same life style. Priorities, values, wants, and, most important, real needs are going to vary among all of us. For example, travel is now very important to me while owning a second home (a cabin in the woods perhaps), doting on children/grandchildren, or having that Catalina 35 may trump travel any day for you. The point here is taking the time to establish where you really need to be with your finances and taking the time to get to that place comfortably, sanely, and relatively stress free. Life—a financially balanced life—is really good and will probably make your later years a heck of a lot more productive and fun!

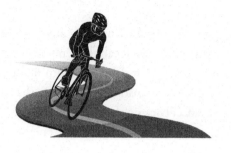

Chapter 14

# *Family and Friends: "Shower the people...."*

This chapter, like others in this book, could be a book in itself. The fact that it consists of only about eight pages must not be regarded as a suggestion from me that it is of lesser importance than other areas of consideration in this discussion. After all, what can beat family and friends in a full, rich life? I think it is precisely our common acceptance of this importance that alleviates the need for a relatively extensive narrative here.

I begin with an important disclaimer relating to family. As you already know, I have no experience in rearing my own children; I do not have any. So, any discussion of family from me comes without the joys and heartbreaks of having my own issue walking among us. That said, I feel confident in noting that I have certainly played an important role in the rearing of at least half a dozen folks who are now in their twenties and thirties, not to mention the hundreds if not thousands of former students and legal clients who are—in a sense—part of my extended family. We'll call them my surrogate children, brothers, and sisters whom I brought into my life as a naval officer and college-level instructor for more than a couple of decades. As I reflect back on these relationships, I realize that I have learned as much or more than I have taught. Additionally I have been given as many or more wonderful gifts than I have given back in my relationships with these folks. Thank you—I have been a very lucky man!

Regardless of how big and/or diverse our immediate or extended family[55] is or how many friends we have, few of us would dispute the importance they have in our lives. I am a great fan of having my own time—alone—to think, to sort things out, to test myself, even to travel—but I also know down to my core that when it comes to my very best experiences, my most memorable times I have virtually always had someone who matters to me to share them with. And that makes all the difference. Sharing life's important and even not-so-important moments and events with those closest to us is—as is the case with all things that make life so wonderful—engaging, fulfilling, exciting, and sustaining. Unfortunately, for some folks, infirmity or despair or hostility brought on by the aging process drives a wedge between them and those who have been closest to them. I have seen this and it is heartbreaking. Let me tell you about such a person; we'll call him Scott. Although you don't know him, you have probably seen someone you do know going through something similar.

---

[55] And, yes, I am going to include the non-human animals that we hold close. Just about all of us have had a family dog or cat or other non-human animal that has lived with or very near to us; if not we know someone who has. The bonds can be extraordinarily close.

I have known Scott for about forty years. When I met him, he was fun and funny, social, attractive, engaged, a Republican although relatively moderate in his political views, in pretty good shape, and hopeful for the future. About a year and a half after we became friends, Scott got married; I was even in the wedding party. Through the years, we did not have many chances to get together and I think it has been about ten years since we last got together. That last meeting was not fun. I found that Scott had become obese—very heavy … and slow. I had learned previously that he had started drinking much more heavily than he used to. He had become harsh, reactionary in his political beliefs, and without any semblance of the sense of humor that was such a joy to those who used to share his company. He was very unkempt and downright unattractive in virtually every way. Needless to say, Scott was enormously unhappy. I supposed he was depressed but both he and his wife (we'll call her Jill) claimed that he was not—even though I never asked about this. During our conversation, I asked Scott if he had heard from this old friend or that one. It was obvious that Scott had "lost touch" with just about all of our old mutual friends and many folks and family members whom he once held close for one reason or another. What was worse, he had not spoken to any of his three children in several years—for reasons that he did "… not care to get into…." If there was a common thread to just about everything we discussed, it was Scott's insistence that he no longer "gave a shit" about what anyone thought about him (or just about anything else, it appeared).

Scott's wife was still pleasant and fairly attractive but she had lost her vitality and she was clearly fundamentally unhappy. Nevertheless, she stayed with him. I am not certain why, but

I guess it was out of commitment or fear of being alone or the effort it would take or all of these things. I was unaware of any major calamity or life-altering issue that had knocked Scott's life for a loop, and he and Jill had a nice home in an affluent neighborhood with no financial problems I was aware of. Both Jill and Scott had excellent retirement benefits. It was clear that the light had gone out of their lives and it was very disturbing and sad to see. It was also clear that this would be our last visit; Scott was obviously uncomfortable around me and made a point of letting me know how much he disliked having his "routine" interrupted; at this, Jill feigned a woeful smile.

I was and still am totally stumped as to why Scott had stopped growing, stopped living. I do know that he had developed a few health issues like arthritis and diabetes, but these are not things that necessarily cause the sorts of major attitudinal and even physical changes that he had obviously gone through. Jill died of cancer a year and a half ago. I sent Scott a note … and then another one … and another. He has not responded. I know that he is still alive only because a neighbor keeps me posted.

What has this sad story to do with aging deliberately? I would say that it has everything to do with it. For specific reasons that I simply do not know, Scott decided—some time ago—to stop growing, to give in, to die inside while still being. I am certain Scott suffered and still suffers a great deal, but he is definitely not alone. Friends and family members of Scott and those like him suffer, as well. What is particularly sad is that there was probably some point when Scott was close to giving up but not quite there yet when someone (possibly me) could have reached out and pulled him back or at least convinced him to see a professional counsellor who could have intervened and possibly helped to prevent the living death of Scott. It didn't happen and Scott is apparently lost to us all. I sincerely believe that many of us have within us the same stuff that took Scott down and away. Call it inertia, emotional ruin, profound sadness, depression, or any or all of these or many other terms we could use, but it is certainly mental illness and it often comes with aging. Our hearts are broken when we see it and I, for one, will always attempt to help friends and family who suffer in this way to seek professional assistance. At the same time, I reach out to close friends and family members when, on those rare occasions, I am feeling down, in pain, or emotionally/mentally exhausted. I am very fortunate to be able to do this and to get a great bounce when I do. For some folks, this is a much more difficult evolution which takes our patience and the help of professionals. The fact of the matter is that we are all in this together. Aging deliberately is a shared experience with those closest to us: celebrating the Wonder of Life and dealing with the setbacks and challenges that aging in it brings.

Heavy stuff, I know. So, let's move on to something a little lighter. I'll do that by asking a question: Is there anything in life better than eating, drinking, playing, traveling, sharing, working, or just being with your friends and family? I think not. Sure, giving love to and receiving love from those close to you will eventually lead to pain when unpleasant things happen to those for whom we care so much. But the wonder and joy of having people we care about close (emotionally if not physically) is the bond that—with Self Love—holds a truly meaningful and rich life together. My close friends and family members are relatively few, but my love for them and dedication to them is boundless. These relationships make me a better person. As a result, I have found that what, as a young man, I expected would happen as I aged is true: Aging deliberately simply cannot become a reality for us without important person-to-person relationships. There don't have to be many. Once again the key is quality over quantity.

Since the really special relationships that we are so fortunate to have in our lives will remain special and even grow in texture and depth if we nurture them, I believe we can be proactive in ensuring that this is exactly what will happen. Here are a few things that I try to keep in mind and put into practice to nurture and grow my relationships with my Family and Friends (especially Barbara) and, consequently, to give and receive the most from those who really matter, those whom I love.

> **Patience**—Remember how you were taught as a child to "count to ten…" before saying anything or responding to some situations. Well, sometimes counting to a thousand and then another thousand is even better. It's really worth it!

> **Tolerance**—This goes hand in hand with patience. It is a key component of kindness.

> **Generosity**—Giving our time, our attention, (occasionally) our money, and our love.

> **Trust**—I sincerely believe that building and maintaining trust is at the foundation of all significant relationships.

**Conversation**—There is no substitute for communicating with those whom we love—especially when we have felt wronged by one or some of them. This is especially important, I believe, in making a habit of going to bed at night at peace, without anger, calm. Talking things out really helps … and you know it. And sometimes it may be wise to seek out a professional since Friends and/or Family may simply be too close to be of help—as much as they want to be. I have received counseling from a professional more than once and I am a better person for it.

**Sincere and timely apologies**—I try not to have reasons to apologize to folks I love for my behavior—crabbiness, inattention, inconsideration, etc.—but when an apology is called for I do not hesitate. It is healthy and helpful!

**Forgiveness**—I saved this for the end of this list because nothing is more important in building and sustaining human relationships—especially the one we have with ourselves—than forgiveness. Anger and hatred consume and poison us—especially, it seems, as we age. The real victim of all of this negativity is not the person who is the object of these feelings. The real victim is the person who harbors the negativity. And, you know something, most of us are well aware of this. The challenge, of course, is to act … to let the bad feelings go—completely, forever. Tough to do in some cases, but oh so good for our lives. So give this a shot. No matter what the source of the negativity may be, work on letting it go. You will live longer and feel better as a result. And you know that, too!

I am certain that you could add one or more things to this list. I encourage you to do so and to let me know what you think that I have left out. What matters most, however, is the thought that we give to how we relate to our Friends and Family—our most essential companions during our lives—while aging deliberately. Now … do yourself a big favor: Find James Taylor's song "Shower the People" and give it a good listen while you reflect on the substance of this chapter. Doing so just might make your day!

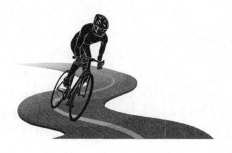

Chapter 15

# *Love and Intimacy: Becoming and Staying Really Close*

I t seems to me that the subject of Love and Intimacy is a natural after our discussion of Family and Friends, so here we go. I think it is fair to say that each of us has a pretty good idea of what love is—regardless of the degree to which we have been able to experience it. That said, philosophers, social scientists, artists, and many others have attempted for millennia to define it and express it. I am going to take a Forrest Gump approach here. You may recall that, during a particularly poignant scene in the movie, Forrest says something simply profound to the love of his life, Jenny, after she appears to have spurned him:

"I'm not a smart man, but I know what love is."

For our purposes, let's not try to over analyze what love is. Let's agree that love is a strong emotion with a deep and intense caring for and/or close identification with someone or something at its core. It's about really really caring for something or someone—a lot. (And, yes, I know that people can love another person but not like them. Noted. Let's move on.)

For most of us, nothing is better than Love. I'm not referring to love of money, success, houses, cars, social status. I am talking about the really important stuff: Love of one's work, spiritual side, friends, family, and, most important, Self. Most of us who have really given some thought to Love would, I believe, agree that unless and until we learn to love ourselves and then nurture that love, we are going to fall short of truly loving all of the other important things and people in our lives. And, if we fall short on loving, we cannot get our heads and hearts completely around aging deliberately. Please don't confuse love of Self with selfishness or narcissism which are rooted in vanity, a self-absorbed and intense admiration of what one has—physical beauty, intelligence, possessions, for example. That type of self-love is not enduring or ultimately fulfilling, and it is most definitely not conducive to aging deliberately. Healthy Self-love is the opposite, really. Self-love allows a person to reach out with kindness, consideration, compassion because the basics are in place. Loving one's Self means that a person has reached an understanding of how to love—a practice involving patience, forgiveness, consideration, compassion, and a certain degree of selflessness, being so at peace inside that there is no longer a need to wallow in worry or to be distracted by doubt and confidence issues. Healthy love of one's Self allows a person's attention to be spent on projecting Self-love outward. It can be a temporary thing or, if a person takes the time to nurture and grow it, it can be enduring.

Like anything that is really important in life, Self-love seems to be both simple and complicated at the same time. It is simple because it focuses only on the important stuff ... and it is complicated because it requires balancing a number of critical components of life—many of which are subjects of various chapters in this book. Most of us can learn to love ourselves, but it does take effort and time. And, once we find that all-important love of Self, we need to pay attention to it, to remain introspective, to continue to grow—not older, but more aware. Of course, balance, once again, is at the heart of this process. If we spend all of our time working on ourselves, obviously there is going to be nothing left for other things and other people. First we get to the point of finding Self-love and then we allow ourselves to grow and develop as needed. With true and lasting Self-love established, time for other things and other people is available and even plentiful. And it is this sharing of the love within that keeps us vibrant, healthy, happy, and fulfilled as we age.

It took me quite a while to get to a point at which I could really love my Self—my string of failed marriages[56] certainly exemplifying my lack of success in this so very important part of life. After lots of introspective thinking, effort, and ... growth, I am there now, and this means that I have the capacity to share love. What a wonder and what a joy!

But just what does loving others[57] mean? What does it entail?

Answering these questions is something that we each have to do in our own way and in our own time. I would

---

[56] More on this later in the chapter.

[57] Not forgetting the extraordinary relations that many of us have or have had with various non-human animals that have added so much to our lives, I am going to focus the love of other human animals for now.

like to call upon a recently acquired friend who helped me to get a better handle on these questions, if not possible answers to them. Within the last year, a friend introduced me to an extraordinarily interesting ninety-year-old man named Bob. Bob is a thinker and a lover—of people. He is also not hesitant to challenge others with great conversation and what Life has taught him. Bob believes that unconditional love—starting with one's Self—is a really good thing, probably something that most of us want, and something that is best achieved by creating our own individual worlds of unconditional love and then projecting outward: "This is my world of unconditional love. You are welcome to join me here. It is entirely up to you because I cannot make you (or anyone else) do anything you do not want to do." To tell you the truth, I don't think this philosophy is quite right for me. Frankly, even though I am quite able and quite eager to forgive—just about anything, I do not forget cruelty, greed, stupidity. Emotional scarring is real and needs to be paid attention to. Continually coming back for more bad behavior, which can often be the case in out-of-balance, enabling relationships, is unhealthy and counterproductive to all-important Self-love.[58]

So ... Bob is an unabashed proponent of unconditional love. I am not—except for my Self-love which I have learned to thoroughly embrace as I continue to nurture it. I have discussed unconditional love of others with the most important person (perhaps ever) in my life, Barbara, whose love for

---

[58] I am not suggesting that my friend, Bob, would advocate this sort of unhealthy relationship vis-à-vis unconditional love—not for a second. I am only making the point to be clear on what I cannot tolerate ... even for a very short time.

her son is, from what I have seen, as deep and intense as any mother's love of child. It exceeds her love for me—any moment of any day—and that is just fine with me. I wouldn't want it any other way. While she is certain that he is incapable of any behavior that could break her tie of love to him, she will concede theoretically, at least, that no love—not even the love of a parent for their children—is truly unconditional. I feel the same way. You see, I now know—for certain—that, while I am more than capable of making mistakes, as long as I am lucid I will never do anything that is unethical, intentionally hurtful, or against my high standards of behavior. I cannot make anyone else live within my own set of living principles, so I am unable to reach that state of absolute trust with anyone else—no matter how much I care about them. I am OK with this, and so is Barbara.

What I can do with my love for others—not just Barbara but everyone I love—is allow it to be as boundless, generous, giving, consistent, and full as I am able. This means no games, honesty (with tact) at all times even when it is difficult to be honest, and openness with my feelings (again with as much tact as is needed). I have not always been able to do this. In fact, this is a relatively recent achievement on my part. Why? Because I used to confuse self-absorption with self-love and, consequently, consistently placed my own momentary comfort and happiness ahead of all others. I don't find it necessary or important to do this anymore. I now can push my immediate needs aside for the sake of focusing on someone else's needs without regret or hesitation or concern that I may be taken advantage of.

You see, I have become extraordinarily comfortable with how I love. I am at peace with it. I no longer worry about how much or how well I love. I just do it. I came to this point in my life—deliberately—through experience, lots of reflection, and effort. Knowing how to love is as wonderful a thing as I have ever known in my life. But … I want to be clear that I am not asking you to embrace my particular loving style. It is not for everyone; it may be for no one else; it may be for most of us. I just don't know, and it is not important. What is vitally important, however, is that each of us gives loving others all the time, energy, and effort that it takes to reach a point where we feel good—really good, way down deep inside—about how we feel about loving others and how we manifest that love each day.

Obviously (I hope) there is a direct tie-in here between love and intimacy. As is the case with many of the terms we are dealing with in these pages, intimacy can mean many different things to many different folks. So, let's see if we can agree on an acceptable definition for our purposes and go from there. I'm going to take a shot by saying that we will consider intimacy as it relates to the special emotional, physical, confidential, possibly even financial relationship between two people who are and wish to remain loving partners indefinitely. These partners are Friends who are Lovers and Lovers who are Friends. Seems like something we can work with; right?

More on the connection between intimacy and aging deliberately in a little while but first—a story, my story—that may shed some more light on the connection between love and intimacy for you as it has for me. You see, I have had more than my share of relationships; I have been through countless attempts to find the final intimate Friend/Lover. Yes, I will go ahead and use the term we have all heard: the Love of my Life. These attempts include five—yes, five—failed marriages[59] which left me thinking that having someone that I really needed[60] in my life was simply not going to happen. Then, owing to serendipity, my own growth (aging deliberately perhaps), and luck, I found Barbara—a close friend of my sister and a woman whom I had known at a distance for about twenty years. Our own prior marriages[61] to and relationships with others had been obvious barriers to our coming together previously. But on Christmas Day 2012, we had a chance to spend some wonderful hours together at my sister's home for family time, dinner, drinks, and lots of fun. I need to tell you this, too: As soon as I saw Barbara walk in the house that day, I was smacked in the head and heart with a feeling that I had never experienced before. I knew that I had finally found my partner for life. Why did everything come together for me at that time and at that place and with this wonderful woman? I have answers but I don't think all of the specifics are particularly relevant here. I will simply say that I was finally ready and able to love and need someone else in a lasting way because my own learning/growing curve regarding my views about myself relative to former partners and my actualization of Self-love made me ready—not for just anyone, but for the beautiful person that Barbara is. The rest I will simply credit to great timing and good old dumb luck on my part. Of course, Barbara did

---

[59] I know this is a shocker … as much to you as it has been—divorce by divorce—to my Friends and Family. And what's more, I was the one who walked away from each one. After my fifth divorce about ten years ago, I really wanted to believe I had finally learned and had grown from what I had been through and had put others through.

[60] Note the distinction here between need and want. This is extraordinarily important to me and goes right to the heart of the linkage between love and intimacy of a lasting sort. In other words, for me, if there is no need for the other person, there can be love but no lasting intimacy.

[61] Barbara has been married once before.

not have a clue at first of what I was feeling. She was initially nowhere near me on this. To make matters more challenging, just a few days later I headed back to my life and job in Florida until the end of January only to begin what was to be a long-planned thirteen-month trip[62] around the world, about fifty countries on all seven continents. Additionally, Barbara was also keenly aware of my relationship/marital history as well as being understandably thoughtful and cautious about the most important things in her life. So … I knew winning her heart would be a slow, deliberate, wonder-full process. She was willing to give me a chance and I was more than willing to be patient. This proved to be a perfect way to start and then to grow. And now … we are together—happy and for Good.

Now for some more on intimacy. I believe that all that applies to love also applies to intimacy—and more. For me at least, as you now know, it is a matter of truly needing in addition to wanting your intimate partner in and for life. And there is still more to it, of course. Despite what dictionaries or common parlance may have to say about intimacy—especially as it relates to physical closeness between two humans who, at least for the moment, have an emotional attachment to each other, I believe intimacy can be shared between family members, to include you and Fido or Felix, good friends, and almost any being (including spiritual ones) to whom we choose to open our hearts. That said, I am going to focus on some thoughts about intimacy between long-time, deeply

---

[62] I knew from the outset that I would return to Michigan (where Barbara lived) for only a couple of weeks during that time. Let's just say, we took advantage of every opportunity to get to know each other better using any methods available—including emails, snail mail, phone calls, and as much time together as time and circumstance would allow.

committed lovers.[63] In doing so, I am going to reach back a bit to something we have already addressed—in the previous chapter. Remember those qualities that I mentioned at the end of that chapter—specifically patience, tolerance, generosity, trust, conversation, sincere and timely apologies, and forgiveness? Yup, I think these are essential to the perpetuation of a truly loving, long-term, monogamous, emotional/physical relationship, and I will have a few additional comments about them a little later in this chapter. But, with respect to love and intimacy, specifically, I would add a few more things: all types of touching (especially kissing), reaching out, always keeping expectations reasonable, and no quid pro quo.

I am a strong proponent of touching, and I think it actually increases in importance as we age. Touching the people I love—especially Barbara—is really easy for me because I am highly tactile at my core. I need and appreciate touching more as I grow, and I like to think that I keep growing every day. I also understand that not everyone is a toucher or likes to be touched—except on occasion. So this section is for those of you who are at least relatively tactile. Hand holding, massaging, kissing, and petting—heavy and less intensely—with a lover are not exclusively within the province of adolescents and twenty and thirty somethings. Madison Avenue generates billions in advertising and sales by selling tactility and sex as a young persons' game. Guess what …. I ain't buying it, and neither should you! Granted, staying in decent physical shape will make us look and feel better and, in turn, may make physical contact more alluring for us and our partners. But, please,

---

[63] To get more involved with all of the possibilities and manifestations of intimacy is the subject for a book, not part of a chapter in a book about aging deliberately.

whatever you do (or don't do) don't be afraid to reach out and touch someone at the right time in the right place. Trust yourself to know when and where …and just do it. Touching is, of course, truly a form of communication. And many forms of communication with those we love can be quite intimate. We all know this. So this is probably a good point to talk a bit more about communication—specifically, reaching out, having and expressing our expectations of others, and just plain talking. First, let's take a look at reaching out.

Some of us or those whom we may love have a tendency to want to withdraw when we feel wronged by someone we love. I used to do that … a lot. It seemed comforting to put up a wall around myself and take comfort in knowing that I could do "just fine" on my own for as long as I wanted—perhaps forever. This is an extraordinarily dangerous thing to do with respect to our relationships with the most important others in our lives. After all, how can we nurture and grow those relationships—an absolute necessity for their maintenance and survival—if we cut them off? This is an excellent point, but when we are hurt and used to withdrawing, it doesn't matter. I know this because I spent a good part of my adult life doing this with the women I supposedly loved. Now, however, my Self-love comes to the rescue and helps me to trust, to need, and … to reach out. This is, of course, the exact opposite of withdrawing. I now find myself able to push aside that reactionary desire to retreat into my own little emotional world when things are not going well with a person I love and to reach out to that person with a sincere desire to be close, to touch, and to talk things out thoroughly, always open to the fact that miscommunication and not an intention to be hurtful is at the root of the issue. And reaching out needs to be done even if you are dead certain that the sole responsibility for the argument or unpleasantness rests with the other person. You see, in such situations fault and blame—not the other person—are the enemies, and reaching out to the other person especially when he or she is defensive and angry is an extraordinarily positive, productive, and loving thing to do.[64]

Another extraordinarily important part of communication which we need to touch upon before getting back to the topic of basic conversation/talking is having and expressing our expectations of others—particularly our lovers. Specifically, reasonable expectations are a necessary part of the most important relationships of our lives (e.g., practicing fidelity, sharing in the creation and development of the home), but unreasonable, subjectively created expectations of our intimate partners (e.g., being ultra-intuitive, responding or reacting to virtually any given situation in a completely predictable fashion) are a major problem in some relationships and can be extremely toxic when consistently tossed into the mix of friendship, love, and intimacy. When others do not live up to our expectations—reasonable or not—we can feel let down, hurt, or even abandoned. But when we find ourselves feeling like this, perhaps the first questions we should ask are whether or not our expectation of the other person was reasonable and … whether it was even known to them. Often the answers to those questions are "No." It seems to me, then, that a key component inherent in avoiding this unpleasant, destructive, and unnecessary issue is doing our best to be sure others know what we expect, to

---

[64] As I mentioned before, if this becomes required in order to sustain a relationship in which one person is always angry or abusive or unwilling to reach out, then it may be time for joint counseling or leaving, since there is obviously no balance in play.

be sure that we make an effort to meet the expectations that have been communicated to us, and to let our lovers know when some expectations cannot be met because they are not reasonable or fair. If, for example, your partner or anyone else whom you love expects you to be enthusiastic about a trip they want to take with you which is very different from anything you have ever done together before and which they said nothing about previously, expectations may be shattered when you respond to the news with little or no interest. Two problems are in play here: the expectation that you would be enthusiastic about this unusual and unexciting trip and your way of responding—especially if it is quick and negative—to the proposal which is obviously very important to the other person. We all know this sort of scenario unfolds between two loving, intimate partners more often than it should. If, however, we are clear and fair with our expectations of others and handle things tactfully and lovingly when expectations—reasonable or not—cannot be met, the potential for serious disappointment and damage to relationships can be drastically reduced.

All of what we have been discussing here can be made infinitely less complicated and a heck of a lot more fun if we simply talk to each other. And, of course, listening carefully is essential. I'm not referring to idle chit chat and banal banter about routine stuff here. That stuff is easy to do and too much of it from one partner or the other can really be annoying. No, I am referring to the occasional heart-to-heart communication about things like interpersonal issues, health concerns, values, sex, children and/or grandchildren, behavior, finances, and, yes, expectations. Consistent, open, fair, considerate conversation between partners in a loving, intimate relationship builds and maintains trust, fosters forgiveness, and minimizes unreasonable expectations. You know the couples who communicate and the ones who—even though they have stayed together for any number of reasons—do not. It is no mystery who is happier and healthier. And try to keep in mind that the process, the actual acts of communicating, of talking, may not always be fun or pleasant. That's perfectly OK. Sometimes reaching an understanding about something important—something that loving couples do not agree on—is challenging, emotionally draining work. But it is good, worthwhile work—a labor of love, if I may—and the rewards are enormous. And, once again, I think this is especially important as we age because it exercises our ability to be reasonable, open, and caring and, in the process, helps us to grow and love as we age—deliberately.

This brings me to yet another critical component of intimacy while aging deliberately with our partners. I discussed it in Chapter 14, but I want to touch on it again here. It is that important, and it's yet another aspect of communicating with your intimate one. I am referring here to the art of the sincere and timely apology. We have all seen it or have experienced it first hand: folks treating those closest to them poorly. Impatience, criticism, intolerance, pettiness… all directed at those we supposedly love most. It seems that some people take their loved one's love and commitment for granted and, unfortunately, this bad behavior often increases with age. I hate to see it and I am very uncomfortable when it happens. But even for those of us who work hard at being sensitive to the feelings of others, the unkind comment, impatience, or unfair criticism may occasionally sneak out and hurt our partners. When it happens, make a point of taking the opportunity to apologize—sincerely and in a timely manner. Please don't let bad acts or language linger. On the other hand, if you feel your partner has been unfair or unkind, let things settle down for a little while, but then do approach your lover/friend and gently tell them how and why you are hurting. I've seen couples practice this—being especially mindful of it as they grow older. It is all about real love, trust, and fairness ... and it works.

Finally, please consider this: Growing and sustaining a healthy, long-lasting intimate relationship is not a matter of quid pro quo. We are at our best when we are kind, patient, considerate, trusting, and generous to others—especially our friend/lovers—when we behave in a truly loving way ... not because that is how we expect to be treated in return but because it is simply the right thing to do. Balance is, of course, extremely important here. If we often find ourselves being on the abused end of a conversation or the day's events or virtually always the one seeking out peace or harmony, it just may be time for professional help and, if that does not work, it may be time for a change. Self-love—the most important love—requires us to respect ourselves, our dignity, and our autonomy in a balanced fashion. We must be willing to be honest enough with ourselves and our partners to recognize abuse of any kind and deal with it in a healthy way. Now ... go give your intimate partner, your Friend/Lover a big hug and a kiss ... and tell them how much you love them.

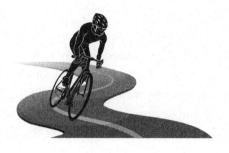

Chapter 16

# Faith and Spirituality: Reaching Out to Something Greater

This is the briefest chapter in the book. As was the case with Chapter 14, however, its length should not, by any means, be regarded as some sort of implication on my part that it is of lesser significance with respect to aging deliberately. Like so many other subjects and chapter titles in this book, it is a critical component of having a really high quality life as we add years to our lives. I am certain that you have already given lots of consideration to what I have to say in this chapter and that is a really good thing. In any case, the topic of spirituality is a must-discuss subject whenever we contemplate living life well, completely.

Faith, spirituality, religion, or whatever word you care to objectify how you reach out to be in touch with Something greater than and beyond your Self is enormously important to many of us. I am going to use the term "spirituality" here so that I can have a term at hand to speak of this without confusing the matter with different terms. And, by the way, I don't think it is important for me to get involved in explaining my views on such things. If you really want to know what *I* think, drop me a line or stop by some time and we'll talk. What I do want to discuss here is the importance of having Something beyond your Self to connect to in some especially important way and how this relates to a full, meaningful life and, ultimately, aging deliberately.

I want to start with a question: What does spirituality mean to *you*? If you haven't given this some serious thought lately, perhaps you should. I am not talking about *practicing* what you believe or thinking about your belief in a detached albeit reverent manner. I am talking about spending considerable effort and energy in thinking about what *exactly* you believe and *why*. It will come as no surprise to any of us that there are plenty of folks who simply believe what they believe because that is what they learned and felt comfortable with as children and that is just the way it is. I suppose that is fine for some of us, but I have come to realize that, for many folks, coming to a real understanding of what and how we believe, through reflection and introspection, is almost as important as belief itself.

About a year ago I had a pretty intense conversation about spirituality with a friend of mine. I knew that he had a very deep and abiding commitment to his faith, but I did not know how intense it was until our conversation. The bottom line for him was that God is Everything to him. I know that many of us have heard similar things about God: God is *in* everything; God is all around us everywhere, every day. But, for my friend,

God is not only in everything all of the time, but God is *the* most important thing to him. God is always central to my friend's plans for the week, his views on everything from art to politics, and even his own life. Spirituality for my friend is, quite simply, God. Now his definition of God is Christianity-based, so Christ is intimately tied in with his faith. But my point here is not to explore *what* spirituality is to my friend. I simply want to acknowledge that, for some folks (perhaps you), spirituality is an extraordinarily intense, personal thing—not *in* Life but *as* Life. My own notions of spirituality are not even in the same world as my friend's, but what I found so amazing about what he shared with me about his belief was how little he actually said about it in our day-to-day interactions. He is a perfect example of a person who can be absolutely committed to his/her spiritual side without being evangelistic, and I, for one, really appreciate that.

On the other hand, I am sure we all know folks who are constantly referring to their faith or the trappings of organized religion. I do not regard this constant professing as spiritual-ity—*unless* it is based on an honest commitment to a life led as consistently as reasonable with the basic tenants of the person's religion. But, even then, I really don't want to have that be the main topic of conversation every time I talk with someone. Please don't misunderstand what I am saying here. This is not an anti-organized religion treatise. As a matter of fact, I truly envy people who have a strong faith in God and/or God's representatives or incarnations on earth. I celebrate the peace and comfort that so many people find in having a close relation with their spiritual side—however it manifests itself. But I also believe spirituality is a personal thing and should never be used as a tool to manipulate, or to harm other non-believers, or to discriminate which, unfortunately, happens just about everywhere every day. I know others who say that they feel the same way, but they still judge those who feel and think differently than they do about things spiritual.

Balanced, personal, genuine spirituality can be the source for most of what is really Good within us. It can be the incentive and/or foundation for incredible acts of kindness, generosity, and love. It can be *the* muse for our creative side and for works of art—great and small. It can help us to be productive at work and to be leaders—in good times and bad. It may be what motivates us to work especially hard at all family and other loving relationships. Our spirituality can help to keep us healthy—physically by guiding diet and exercise and psychologically/emotionally by providing guidance and answers to the most difficult questions confronting us in our human experience. For many of us, spirituality can also be *the* source of comfort during times of suffering, illness, and loss—*especially* as we age and lose capacities, loved ones, and, eventually, our own worldly lives. Moreover, spirituality is, I believe, any or all of these things ... and more.

Perhaps this is really the essence of what spirituality really is: a servant to our Selves and the quality of our Lives which is best experienced if we actually serve *it* through what we think and do each day. However you have found or come to find spirituality, my guess is that how you feel or what you think about in relation to what I have said in this chapter—whether you think that it makes sense or not—has been reinvigorated. And, since spirituality is so utterly important in aging deliberately, I will acknowledge that importance by avoiding further, possibly distracting discussion by closing here. Namaste.

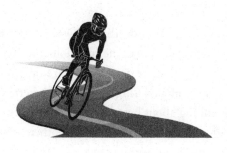

Chapter 17

# Contemplating Death: Becoming Comfortable with and Prepared for The End

"It is better to travel well than to arrive."[65]

I am on a long flight from Seoul to Dallas as I write this. It is late; no one is stirring. The only sound in the cabin is the moderate white noise of the jet engines. I feel alone, but not lonely, and I have just reread my chapter about spirituality. This is an excellent time and place to share with you some of

---

[65] I know that you know that this quotation is really not attributable to the Buddha. Most folks who look into these kinds of things think its closest parent is "To travel hopefully is a better thing than to arrive [from an essay by Robert Louis Stevenson entitled "El Dorado," 1878]." For me, it is not important who first said it or when it was first uttered. I simply love the concept, and it seems to me to be an exceptionally upbeat way to begin a chapter on Death. It also just happens to be reminiscent of my own views on travel—as reflected in the title of my first book: *Traveling Deliberately*. (Not plugging here…just connecting the dots on an idea.)

my contemplations about death. And when I refer to death in this chapter, I am referring to the cessation of the breath taking and heart beating that we do while we are in this life on this earth. I am not contemplating death as a theoretical subject or state. I am talking about being dead and the state of our own individual deadness ... not the deaths of others whom we may know or not or whom we may love or not. My guess is that we will find lots of common ground on this—especially since you have stayed with me this long and we have become fellow travelers to at least some degree.

Don't you think that death is not quite as big a deal as some would make it? Sure, if we are up against something life threatening—disease, a traumatic injury, life-threatening emergency—we may react in some highly emotional or significantly energized fashion. But I think this is more a matter of Self-preservation than a real fear of death. And I do think there is a big difference between the two. When you really think about it, you may feel as I do that there are only a few things out there to fear: for me, this very short list includes losing my critical thinking faculties and finding it impossible to get around even with the assistance of others. So ... I do whatever I can to stay healthy mentally and physically and let the rest go as best I can.[66] So why don't we simply agree to come to an understanding among ourselves that it is probably much better and healthier to understand death and dying and to prepare for it accordingly than it is to fear it?

Now then, what you thought about in response to what I had to say in the previous chapter about spirituality is probably going to have a huge impact on your thinking about and

---

[66] Once again, the "Serenity Prayer"—so simple and yet so profound—comes to mind.

ultimate understanding of death. Regardless of one's concept and/or practice of spirituality, one thing all rational people can agree on is that this body/mind/spirit package that we currently operate with is, for one reason or another, going to give out on us, and this unit of ours is going to cease to exist in its current state. In short, we—all of us—are going to die. It's OK. I know that the D word has been a huge issue—perhaps the ultimate issue—for generations upon generations of humans, but let's try to take a different approach.

Some folks are so fearful of death or perhaps forgetful of its certainty that they let their fear or their forgetfulness—very egocentric when you think about it—get in the way of the other important people in their lives. Lovers, friends, sons and daughters, siblings … all those close to us are going to have a tough time of it as we near death and/or when we die—perhaps suddenly. Let's not make it more difficult by leaving them to make trying decisions at the most emotionally stressed and, consequently, the worst possible time. Let's take them off the hook emotionally, legally, financially, and ethically by being explicit about our love for them as well as our wishes about our estates, our final healthcare decision-making, our remains—well in advance.[67]

---

[67] This one is especially important to me … and it should be to you. One of the single most environmentally unfriendly decisions a person can make—and I am including many of those folks who think of themselves as environmentally aware here—is to request a traditional funeral and burial. Yes, I am talking about pumping all that nasty toxic goo into one's veins, using all those chemicals on the face and hair to make a person look good, "natural." (Really? Natural?!) The person is dead for crying out loud! Using all of those materials to put together a beautiful coffin that is actually a piece of furniture for a corpse—complete with a soft, comfy, satiny interior, and on and on so that what is created is a mini-hazmat area—is nuts. Even the traditional final preparations for a person who is going to be cremated are an unnecessary, inefficient way of handling things. I could go on and on, but that is not my

And when I say making our wishes explicit, that means in writing: wills, living wills, codicils, etc. This means we have to plan on and for our deaths, and the more/better we do this the less difficult our passing will be on those whom we love. These preparations are going to take some work and maybe even some money but, first and foremost, they are going to take the willingness to accept the fact that we are all going to be goners someday. Being in denial won't help; nor will putting things off just because we may still be in great shape or even be relatively young (in our thirties, forties or fifties). BANG! Never saw that cement truck coming!!

I think the cement truck is a key metaphor that I hold close for a more practical philosophy of death as it relates to aging deliberately. It goes something like this. I am having a really good time in this Life and I believe that my existence in this Life is also making things better for a certain number of human and non-human animals, education, and—in a tiny, tiny way—the environment. Additionally, I have no clue of what, if anything, will follow my current life form. Consequently, I want to do everything reasonably possible to live as high quality of a life[68] as possible for as long as possible. In other words, I am really enjoying the excellent traveling in this Wonder-full journey of my Life. Getting to

---

purpose here. My purpose is this: Consider giving back—even in death—by seeking out an environmentally friendly disposal of your remains. One example is to have them mingled with a seedling tree which can be visited and nurtured in a loving way by generations after you. What a way to age, die, and then linger in a different state as the key ingredients of another living thing! There is a lot more information about this and many other options via the Green Burial Council and many other sources. Please give this some thought.

[68] Simply stated, this means giving and taking really Good things in a Balanced way—each day.

my ultimate destination in this existence (i.e., being d-e-a-d) is something that I would just as soon wait on—especially since I am fortunate enough to be in excellent physical, emotional, and mental condition.[69] So, I will continue to love and to be loved, to eat well, to keep my weight where it should be, to use the supplements that my wellness docs and I agree will best suit me, to exercise, to get plenty of good quality sleep, to think, and—this one is HUGE—to pay attention. You see, paying attention, gets us just about everything: noticing the beauty and the Wonder that is everywhere by using all of our senses—tasting, hearing, seeing, smelling, touching, feeling, or any of these that we have not lost for some reason. At the same time, paying attention (i.e., keeping the totally unnecessary distractions like cell phones, texts, iPods, etc. to an absolute minimum) will also keep us aware and in touch with everything around us—including that cement truck that just crossed the center line (very possibly because its driver is being distracted by a cell phone conversation) and is heading straight for us!

As you can see, my view of my inevitable death is informed by the way I want to (and, in fact, do) live my life. Contemplating death as an end, although maybe not *the* end, of Steve Bannow is a healthy way to appreciate each day—always knowing that death is out there somewhere but also knowing that there are lots of ways of decreasing the odds that today will be the day that you get the visit.

---

[69] Again … no attempt on my part to be glib here. I am fully aware that a serious permanent disruption in the state of my current physical, emotional/mental condition could change my feelings about this. But hear me out and see how what I still have left to say speaks to this concept of preserving generally excellent health and, thus, the desire to keep moving forward as long as possible.

When you think about it, if you have been living your Life fully and you have been aging deliberately by caring, being responsive, paying attention (to everything),[70] and moving forward despite the challenges that will inevitably confront us, is there really any time to fear death or to even worry about it? I think that the answer is an emphatic NO! And I know that a healthy understanding of and preparation for death can only make Life more special.[71]

---

[70] And this includes taking time to prepare for every death and dying issue, environmentally sound body disposal directives, life insurance policies, wills, legacies, living wills, etc.

[71] I know of no one who gets this death business better than President Jimmy Carter. He was recently diagnosed with what very well could be terminal cancer. He has been strong, classy, humble, positive, graceful, and very public about his illness. Sure, he is ninety-one, but he still enjoys each day of his life with great vigor, energy, positive thought, productivity, action, and joy. He wants to live just as much as you or I do. What a role model he has been and continues to be!

# Conclusion

It is the end of April and I have just returned to my home in Michigan after a ten-week trip to Hawaii, New Zealand, Australia, and seven countries in Asia. It was a very active adventure, and I was pretty well spent by the time I left Seoul, South Korea, my last stop. The eleven-and-a-half hour flight to Dallas was, by no means, the longest flight that I have ever taken, but it did me in. Twenty-four hours after I had landed in Detroit I was feeling really rocky … for good reason: I had picked up a case of pneumonia. These events make *now* a perfect time to write the conclusion to this book about aging deliberately. Why would I say that?

Up to this point, I have focused on the positive … with lots of perky quips on movement, staying active—mentally, emotionally, and physically—being positive, paying attention, being in the moment, getting all that we can out of each day, loving avidly. It would *seem* like I am the Energizer Bunny—constantly up, never slowing down, always ready for something new, looking for additional (and fun) new challenges at every turn. The truth of the matter is that, like anyone else, I have my down times—especially when I am sick. And … when I am down, I often find myself asking if what I did previously to being burned out, or ill, or exhausted to the bone was actually worth the price. What was I *thinking*?! Why did I *do* that? I should have *known* that last trip or adventure was going to be (too) difficult. (Note all of the italics!) In fact, over the last several days—while fighting chills, fever, a terrible cough, nasty aches and pains, serious exhaustion—I found myself asking these very same questions. My point is that I was down hard ... and I knew it. So, the key question then becomes: When we *do* hit the deck, what do we do in response? And why does this matter—especially as we move into our forties, fifties, sixties, and beyond? Kind of a provocative way to wrap up my thoughts about this aging deliberately business, if I do say so myself!

I find that it is especially challenging for those of us who are fortunate enough to enjoy extraordinarily good health and to maintain a pervasive perkiness (that, to some, may seem to border on perpetual mania) to be sick, to lack energy, to be physically run down to the point of being not interested in doing just about *any*thing. But, I assure you, it happens. As I suggested above, I have been dealing with this very issue for the past ten days. What I have done to sustain myself and to stay positive is to be mindful that this state is *temporary*. It is *not* the beginning of the end; it is *not* a "sign" that I am now supposed to permanently switch gears and move into a new, slower routine; it was and is time to heal—to accept that sickness, down days, and the need for a temporary break in the action to rest and recover do enter our lives occasionally. And I, for one, am good with this and thankful, gleeful that what hit me has been nothing more serious or permanent. So ... I have learned acceptance in this regard and with this, I understand how acceptance is essential for healing and how healing leads to the road to recovery and, ultimately, to live the active, full, deliberate Life that I have grown to love and appreciate.

Now that I am in the recovery mode—I'm at about seventy-five percent at this point thanks to plenty of rest, love from Barbara, and some kick-ass antibiotics—I have been taking time to give some thought to what, if anything, I have *learned* or *should have learned* as a result of this last bout of illness. I started with something positive. I (re)learned something I already knew: Know yourself well enough to know when you really *do* need medical attention—*and seek it out ... promptly ...* as I did this time. I didn't know that I was as sick as I was, but I *did* know that I needed help. I received it and I did not get worse. I am healing now. I learned something new, as well. If I do return to certain Asian countries—and big-cities in China, in particular—I will give serious consideration to wearing one of those surgical masks made famous by our Japanese friends. One huge reason is air pollution. The air quality in Delhi and Beijing and many other large metropolitan areas in India and China really is not good and the mask will keep a lot of that bad stuff out of the throat and lungs. Also, it stands to reason that really bad air causes lots of sneezing, coughing, and hacking among the folks who live and work and play in it. Lots of these folks simply do not cover properly when their body fluids come flying out—often times on my shoulders, neck, and, yes, even my face. I am not going to apologize for being graphic here. I am simply telling how it is and what I have learned and what I am likely to do in response—*if* I return. I am certain that I have/will have learned more about myself and my life as I reflect on my last low period, but I think my point about *continuing* to learn and grow from life's experience—*forever*—has been made.

Learning's most important sibling is *growth*. Growth is a really, really Good thing and perhaps the most important component of aging deliberately. Remember my mantra and the key theme of this book: We do not *grow* old; we *become* old because we *stop* growing? Growth is the putting into action of what we learn from living. It moves us on ... ahead. It is the substance of a rich, ever-improving, deliberate life. Growth is the essence of tomorrow's promise. If you ever doubt the importance of growth, just think of where each of us individually and all of us collectively would be without it—stasis, a void, repetition. Learning and consequential growth as a result of our down time is smart; it is almost like learning from failure—so important since we so rarely learn from success or become permanently stronger from living in the status quo.

A significant portion of what I have had to say so far in this conclusion has been philosophical .... So what, in a more practical sense, is there to do when we falter because of a physical set back or—perhaps even more challenging—a psychological one?[72] I think the really tough thing is—when the opportunity presents itself ... and, whether we realize it at the time, or not, it will—to get back in the proverbial saddle and start to ride again. [73]

It's not the speed or style of the ride that matters; it's all about the ride itself. This often means pushing aside sometimes huge physical and emotional baggage—inertia, hatred, anger, fear—and taking the chance to get back to what truly

---

[72] The death of a loved one perhaps or dealing with the psycho-emotional side of some other type of permanent loss—a limb, one's hearing, the family homestead, for example.

[73] Lest I appear to be too glib here, let me hasten to add, once again, that *loss*—mind-numbing, paralyzing loss with accompanying clinical depression—is out of my league and way beyond the reach of this discussion. Depression is serious mental illness and—no matter what its source—requires professional evaluation and treatment far beyond the anecdotal, self-help, you-can-do-this sorts of insights and advice that I am offering in these pages. Depression is far too complicated and serious a condition to be taken on alone. If this is a concern for you or a loved one, try to take the initial, almost always most difficult first steps to find the help you or your loved one need.

fulfills us, makes us happy, and keeps us moving … ahead, deliberately. We all have read or heard wonderful stories of inspiration in which someone is confronted by a seemingly impossible-to-overcome challenge. Something inside that person pushes her to risk everything to move on, to move ahead. Is that "something" will or ego or spirit or Life itself? I assure you that I don't know exactly what it is or if it is the same thing for each of us. I do believe—profoundly—however, that each of us has at least some spark of "it" inside of us. (Otherwise, we would be dead.) And it is what we *choose* to do with it—even during the most challenging times—that does not measure our quality as individual human beings but most assuredly *does* measure the quality of our existence.

This is just the right place for me to relate a story about a person whom I have known for a very long time who exemplifies the high-quality-of-life seeking tenacity that I have been talking about—in this chapter, specifically, and throughout all of these pages, generally. There are, however, a couple of big challenges in trying to do this. The first one is that everyone who reads this book is either such a person or knows one, so whatever I have to say may be relatively unnecessary to connect the dots and complete my point. Another challenge is that I have known more than just a couple of folks who have managed to hang in there and enjoy high-quality lives despite facing all kinds of things that might make others of us give in or give up. I am going forward with this anyway. What I have to say here just may conjure up really Good connections with the people in your lives who have made you cry with Wonder and love as they moved forward—despite being dealt a really nasty hand. I have chosen to tell you about this particular person because, frankly, I need to write about her.

The central character in the story (for now, we will refer

to her as E) lost her mother, her husband, and, in a sense, one of her children in a period of about ten years. Each loss came after an enormous amount of selfless giving and caring for each ... all while working a full-time job and raising a family. E's Hubby (we'll call him M), whose story is also beyond inspirational, turned what he was told would be "... a few months of life full of suffering ..." into two-and-a-half-plus high-quality years of Life. I'll have much more to say about M later.

E's mother started dying in 1973—the year her husband died and she chose to continue to smoke cigarettes. E's mother was a loving, once active person whose emphysema would eventually become an extraordinarily complicated mixture of life-threatening and quality-of-life ending conditions. Yet E found a way to do just about everything anyone could think of to love, care for, and spend time—lots of time—with her mother to make like life as good as it could be, especially during the last two to three years. By the way, M was exceptionally supportive during these days and certainly did his own superb loving and care-giving to E's mother. By the time E's mother finally died in 1985—her heart still beating hours after her lungs completely ceased to function—E was completely spent, but never—not once—complained about what she was going through or had experienced while doing all that she could to care for and comfort her mother. E was not vying for sainthood; this is just how she rolled and still does today.

Within three years of losing her mother, her dearest Friend and the most cherished person in her life—her hubby, M—was diagnosed with a very aggressive form of liver cancer which was rapidly moving through his body. He was told that he had a few months to live and that none of his few remaining months were likely to be the least bit pleasant for him. This is where Team E and M kicked into gear. Providing the details of how they moved forward and fought back—together as mates and fantastic parents—is a book in itself (one which E herself may wish to write at some point … sure hope so). We will say, for starters, that a prognosis of a very unpleasant few months of unhappy life culminating in a miserable death was simply … unacceptable to E and M. Their pushback started with research and consultations. No type of treatment was to be ruled out without close scrutiny. M went through chemo and radiation therapy; together they sought alternative treatment in Mexico; they went to an entirely organic vegetable juice diet for M; and they also brought many other positive practices (such as channeling, lots of exercise, and plenty of opportunities for Family love, and laughter) into play. I knew this couple well and I can tell you that what I witnessed them endure—individually and as a couple—was almost beyond belief. And again … virtually entirely without one complaint or "poor me." Life was simply too dear, too important for anything but positive movement forward.

On a mid-September day, more than two-and-a-half years after M was diagnosed, the battle, the movement, and the life for the couple ended. I presided at M's memorial service. The entire world was there. It was a celebration of a Life extraordinarily well lived. M's oldest son and I went out later that night. Taxis were involved. I'll let it go at that.

Within a few years of M's death, one of E's children, who was going through significant emotional and sociological issues, decided to reject E. Family dynamics will not allow me to divulge the specifics here. I will sum up a significant component of the story by saying that a certain domestic relations court judge made a shocking final ruling that greatly exacerbated the already difficult situation. The judge's motives, legal principles, and ethics behind that ruling defy rational explanation to this day. Consequently, the child was lost—at least for the time—to E. This one just about crushed her, yet she found a way to move forward—always knowing (as mothers do) that the current state of affairs was, by no means, the real end of their relationship. As it turned out, after a very difficult period for all involved and hard lessons learned by some, the family healed itself and became whole again—largely because E simply would not give up on preserving her family. Tenacity and forgiveness make a formidable duo in such matters.

During that same time period, E lost her balance on a patch of ice on a very cold winter's day and fell. In the process, her ankle was fractured in a grotesque way. After several surgeries and a tremendous amount of therapy, she was finally able to walk. That ankle, however, was wrecked and continues to cause E lots of trouble to this day. Nevertheless, E has found a way to remain active, upbeat, attractive, and … moving forward.

So what exactly is "the way" that E found (and that M found) to hang in there, to remain positive, to Live despite loads of personal challenges and heartache? I will never know and neither will E. I am sure that each of us would jump at the chance to bottle up "the way" and give it to anyone who wants it. My best guess is that somewhere along the way each of us makes a choice about how we will deal with all of the Good and terrible things that will inevitably find a way into our lives. Obviously, E and M's choice was focused on the conviction that quality of Life is extraordinarily important, essential. Consequently, they made a commitment to keep moving forward, making each day truly a special gift. They were inspirational. Although never having been challenged the way E and M have been, I have made the same choice and so has Barbara whose own story is an extraordinary profile in courage and strength and positivism.

By now, you have doubtless figured out that the thinly disguised E and M of my story are my sister, Elissa, and my brother-in-law, Mike. Why not? They were and continue to be inspirational to me and to everyone who knows/knew them—as, to a small extent, you also now have had the good fortune to.

What I have learned from Elissa and Mike and Barbara and others like them is life altering and life expanding. Consequently, all I had to do was to pay attention, to learn, and to grow. I owe these folks more than I can ever tell them, but I can live in a way that keeps in motion their wonderful examples. So … for me, the process during my recent down time has been a matter of accepting but not giving in to my physical illness. Let's not minimize the accompanying psycho-emotional hit that is so often a part of something like this. I know that getting the medical attention I need, along with making the necessary adjustments in my daily routine, will get me back to the level of health that I so enjoy. I find myself making a point of keeping the importance of learning and growing as a result of these down days at the forefront. I do this while preparing for the time when—as gradual as it may be—I will need to get back in the saddle. And getting back in there for me is a combination of mental activity (such as finishing this book), physical activity (slowly getting back to my full work-out schedule), and cooking and eating in a well-rounded, healthy manner. (This last component is especially important for me since I have lost about ten pounds over the last two or three weeks taking me down to about 152 pounds which, at six feet one, is not a healthy weight for me, to say the least.) I am working—actively, consciously—through this process. And I will tell you something else: It has not been easy. Between the pneumonia and the rot-gut, kick-ass antibiotics I have been taking, I have felt absolutely terrible at times over the past ten days or so. As I mentioned previously, however, I have been sustained by the knowledge that being down is temporary and that I would grow, learn, and endure even if it were not. And then ... there is the truly amazing power of laughter. I have resorted to humor and laughter often during this period—especially when I have been at my worst—and I have experienced significant progress as a result.

I have been a fan of both self-deprecation and laughing at adversity—especially my own—since my own mental/intellectual coming of age in my mid-twenties. No one in my experience, however, better used the power of laughter more effectively in truly grave circumstances than my best friend and brother-in-law Mike, who learned it or at least refined his awareness of it by reading what Norman Cousins and others had to say about the curative effects of laughter, of humor. Norman Cousins ultimately died at the age of seventy-five in 1990—thirty-six years after being diagnosed with severe heart disease—but, like my brother-in-law, found a way through pain and setbacks by being able to find ways to laugh. Obviously, Norman Cousins and my brother-in-law made it through some very difficult times with their own acute and chronic health issues—issues that make mine pale in comparison—but the point has not been lost on me and should not be lost on you ... even if you are down really hard right now. Allowing ourselves an opportunity to find humor in life and to laugh—hard ... is really good for us. For example, in response to what watching Marx Brothers' films did for him while fighting an especially difficult debilitating, potentially lethal bout of his chronic disease, Cousins reflected:

I made the joyous discovery that ten minutes of genuine belly laughter had an aesthetic effect and would give me at least two hours of pain-free sleep. When the pain-killing effect of the laughter wore off, we would switch on the motion picture projector again and, not infrequently, it would lead to another pain-free interval.

Not only did looking for and appreciating humor—and especially unbridled laughter—in life add years to Norman's, Mike's, and many others' time on earth but, perhaps more important, it greatly increased the quality of their lives. I love that, am strengthened by it, and have done lots of growing—especially over the last ten years or so—by paying attention to it.

It certainly is not my intention to spend all of my space in this Conclusion on illness, what it is like to be off our respective games, and what positive things we can do to get back on track. I think that you probably got the point some paragraphs or even pages ago. I do, however, want to be certain that I link what Tom and I have had to say throughout this book about the immeasurable importance of maintaining a healthy, positive attitude even when it seems virtually impossible to do so. After all, to do something deliberately—whether it is working, traveling, or even aging—takes engagement … lots of it. And it is virtually impossible to be truly engaged in something if we are negatively distracted. This is where the dots all start getting connected. When we tend to stay in a generally positive state, we tend to stay engaged. When we are engaged, we pay attention—to the world, to those we love (and those whom we don't), to events, and to our Selves.

Let me give you an example. As you know by now, I really love being active and finding all kinds of new ways to challenge myself physically as well as intellectually. I also pay attention and want my own traveling—metaphorical and literal—to go on for as long as I can. I have had knee issues since I was fourteen (with five operations on my right knee). That knee became a real liability and has been one for years; the pathology calling for a new one had been in place for a long time. So, in the late spring of 2014, I made my move. I saw a bone and joint surgeon (Dr. William R. Lee) to have an assessment. I was immediately impressed by Dr. Lee's demeanor and professionalism. He told me that he could go in and "clean it out" (a term that anyone with chronic knee issues and resultant surgeries is well aware of), but that he no longer did that sort of nominal procedure. He further related pretty much what I already knew: I would want a new knee at some point and he would wait for me to tell him when. He was very impressed when I informed him that I had recently finished a trip to Machu Picchu using the very challenging Inca Trail and that I had been involved in some other very challenging physical activity in other parts of South America and Antarctica, including mountain climbing. Dr. Lee noted that I was one of only a tiny fraction of people who could do what I had done considering the state of my knees. When my appointment was nearing its end, I thanked Dr. Lee for his candor and told him I was not ready yet. He nodded in agreement and smiled. We also agreed that I would come back to see him when it was time. Soon after completing the trip I mentioned in this conclusion's first paragraph, I made an appointment to go back to see Dr. Lee. It was time and I was ready. I am ready. As the surgery date grew closer, I noticed that I was not the least bit apprehensive about the procedure.

It was the right thing to do, the timing was perfect, and I knew it because I had been paying attention.[74]

You see, when we are paying attention, we are more likely to notice changes in and issues related to just about everything. Sometimes these changes and issues might relate to our own physical, mental, and/or emotional state. When we are able to notice these things, we give ourselves the opportunity (the choice) *to respond*, not *to react* (which indicates fear and/or panic). Responding demonstrates a desire to know and to move ahead in a positive way with whatever the next step should be. The issue is given the attention that it deserves—in plenty of time before things have gotten out of hand. And with professional help, some luck, and a positive outlook, in all likelihood the problem will be resolved or dealt with in a helpful manner. Life, we hope, will go on in as wonderful a way as it had been going on … and the Wonder-full journey will continue.

You are still with Tom and me after over two-hundred pages, so my guess is that you have found things in this book that have totally baffled you … but the mystery or oddness has kept you reading. Perhaps you have found yourself nodding in agreement with some things that you knew already or perhaps that are new to you and make sense. Perhaps you may have even found something within these pages and that you are likely to think hard about and possibly incorporate into your life in the future. Whatever you do, I hope that you find a way to keep smiling, keep paying attention, and keep moving ahead. After all, aging deliberately really is a good way to go regardless of your starting point.

Take good care of yourself and keep in touch.

---

[74] As I write this, it is post-op day twenty. I am delighted to report that I am enjoying a first-rate recovery as I plan for my next series of adventures on two good knees.

# *Appendix I*

I am going to tell you something that means a lot to me and my attempts to age deliberately. It may be a mildly interesting anecdote for some of you, or it may be a close-to-home story that has huge significance for others. In any case, it deals with attitude, limitations, Self-love, acceptance, growth, and several other important subjects touched upon within these pages.

I was born with a genetic physical anomaly called pectus excavatum (essentially, a caved-in chest). My father had a very mild physical manifestation of it; mine was much more pronounced. It can be detectable at birth or can remain hidden until puberty. I really don't remember much about my condition until I was about twelve. I'm quite sure it did not become particularly noticeable until then. In any case, my chest became an enormous issue for me as I entered seventh grade—with sports, gym class, and lots of time shirtless in showers and playing basketball. It was bad enough that I was painfully aware of how I looked and how different I was than every other boy in my grade and at my entire junior high school or the rest of the world—for all I knew. But it was even worse. Some of the guys in gym class made a big deal about it and—get this—even the two gym teachers (also my basketball coaches) made a point of pointing it out to me and others. I was wary of slow dancing with girls at parties and school dances for fear of their … noticing. Even the thought of someone unintentionally touching me in the chest and finding little there but a sizeable indentation was enough to make me keep my distance.

I think most of us can relate to the awkwardness, anger, pimples, sudden sexual awareness, and other hormone-related issues—or should I say hassles—associated with puberty/early adolescence. In fact, many of us may have stories—some rather funny … now—about things we may have done, felt, or said during this time of our lives. But, for me, there was nothing funny about how I looked and—even now—my experiences, perceived inadequacies, and even self-loathing are a source of some pain. By about the time of my sixteenth birthday, it became clear to me and—thank goodness—to my father that something had to be done.

To his credit, my father did some basic research and scheduled an appointment for me to see a doctor at the University of Michigan Medical School/hospital. The doctor recommended that we see a Dr. Barrett who operated out of Harper Hospital in Detroit. The visit to Dr. Barrett was enormous for me. He was a big guy, an orthopedic surgeon with huge, strong hands. He was kind, funny, and sensitive to what I had been going through. He explained that corrective surgery could be performed and that he had had some good results in the recent past but that there could be no guarantees. I didn't care. I was all in. The summer of 1967 saw my acquisition of my driver's license, horrible rioting in Detroit not far from Harper Hospital while I was recovering from surgery, and a newly reconstructed chest.

My new chest was by no means perfect when all was said and done, but the surgery had been a *huge* improvement.

Despite enduring a great deal of pain and lying in bed with my chest in traction for weeks, I never regretted a moment of what I went through; Dr. Barrett was my hero and I felt like I had become a new, different, *better* person. The challenge did not end with the surgery and post-op recovery and rehabilitation. About a week after getting out of the hospital and a couple of weeks before the beginning of my junior year of high school, I came down with an extremely serious case of pneumonia and was given about a 55-45 chance of pulling through. I obviously did survive and sailed ahead.

I wanted to relate this story because it is something important that will help you to get to know me in this very personal discussion of some of the key experiences of my life as I have grown and aged. It is also a way for me to let you know that I do understand why some of us choose to undergo things in our lives that just need attention—in one way or another. Perhaps, when all is said and done the key question is Tom's question: Are you better today than you were yesterday? Obviously "better" can be interpreted many ways, but the question is always worth asking. I hope your life is full of "yes" answers and that this book is something you can rely on to make that happen.

# *Appendix II*

| Supplement | Benefit | When |
|---|---|---|
| Aspirin (children's) | Heart health, protection against stroke, cancer | Morning |
| CoQ10 (aka Ubiquinol) | Heart health, other support | 2X per day |
| Fish Oil/Omega 3 (also Krill) | Energy, cell building, brain support | 2X per day |
| Glucosamine | Joint support, arthritis | 2X per day |
| Magnesium | Sleep aid, gentle laxative | Bedtime |
| MSM | Joint support, arthritis | 2X per day |
| Multivitamin | Virtually none | For me, never |
| Resveratrol | Anti-oxidant, telomere support | Morning |
| Vitamin B Complex (B1, 2, 3, 5, 6, 12 and folic acid | Energy and anti-toxins | 2X per day, morning and afternoon |
| Vitamin C | Energy and anti-toxins | 2X per day, morning and afternoon |
| Vitamin D3 | Prevention of cancer and dementia, heart and bone health, sleep aid | Bedtime |
| Vitamin K | Normal blood clotting, bone and heart health | Bedtime—especially effective taken with D3 |

# *Index*

CPSIA information can be obtained at www.ICGtesting.com
Printed in the USA
BVOW08s1906290316

442202BV00001B/1/P